THE POWER DIET

Double Your Energy - Boost Brain Power
Supercharge Immunity - Lift Libido
Shed Fat and Feel Amazing!

With 10-Minute Meals
That Taste Like Heaven

Chad Scott

www.ChadScottCoaching.com

Introduction

A little over 20 years ago I awoke to a wrenching pain in my gut that had me crawling to the bathroom. While the pain seemed to mimic common signs of food poisoning (a sharp knife jabbing at my kidneys), I hadn't ruled out the possibility of some merciless virus declaring war on my immune system.

Like most guys, I was raised to be a "real man" and more often than not, encouraged to "tough it out."

Unfortunately (or perhaps, fortunately) after I endured a full three days of consistent vomiting without ever ingesting any food, I realized something was really wrong.

I remember saying to myself, "Hey, this isn't normal and you need to call for help." Eventually, the will to survive overrode my false bravado and I called my mother to take me to the hospital.

After running a cat scan, x-ray, blood test, and several other not so fun invasive protocols, the doctors simply said, "We don't know what it is" and told me to go home and drink lots of fluids.

This whole episode was vexing for me. At the time, I wasn't exactly dining at McDonalds or snacking on Snickers and Coke. In fact, I was eating (at least I thought I was eating) pretty healthy foods like fruits, vegetables, whole grains, fish, chicken and occasionally beef.

Regardless, I continued to consistently get sick. And when I say consistently, I mean consistently.

For instance, instead of looking back on the year and noting how many sick days I had (like most people), I would recount the 10-15 days of the year where I actually felt good. The rest of the days I spent battling some type of cold, virus or inexplicable illness.

Naturally, this downgraded my professional work as I found myself too tired, weak and distracted by pain to actually get much done.

As a lifetime athlete, who once reveled in the joy of sports and the great outdoors, I found myself struggling with constant fatigue as if I was carrying an invisible backpack full of rocks on my back which siphoned off my power supply.

Even my relationships suffered in some not so flattering ways. Literally, flatulence from a bloated gut created constant agitation and discomfort, which made it difficult to sleep next to my partner.

To eliminate the pain and restore my power as quickly as possible my Doctor told me to guzzle some Pepto-Bismol or pop some Advil or take an antibiotic, which only made things worse. Turns out, antibiotics wipe out both good and bad bacteria and can make you more susceptible to illness.[1][2] Antacids kill off valuable stomach acid that helps you digest your food and fight off pathogens.[3][4] And the overconsumption of NSAIDs can blow gaping holes in your gut and lead to peptic ulcers, weight gain, obesity and leaky gut syndrome.[5][6][7]

Of course, my next move was to take the natural route by experimenting with various herbal remedies, which did give me some noticeable relief. Regardless, there was one big monumental challenge with all of these solutions: none of them addressed the root of the problem!

The pills and even the herbs were like band-aids, which only worked short-term - kind of like hacking at the branches of a weed and expecting the root to die. What I couldn't quite figure out was what was causing the root of my power drain.

I kept asking myself if I was cursed with low immunity and a digestive system that didn't work so well? Did I have too much stress in my life, was I overworking myself or was there something else I was missing?

As a Master Results Coach who helps people for a living my natural response was to take a deep dive into the problem and find the answers. Over the course of 20 years of intense study and experimentation I found some remarkable discoveries as well as some perplexing statistics that clearly pointed to some very troubling facts.

Let's just take overeating and the result of being overweight or obese as an example. According to the World Health Organization, obesity worldwide has nearly tripled since 1975 with nearly two billion people who are now overweight.[8] And in the US alone, according to the CDC

(Center For Disease Control), 42% of Americans are obese, which combined with being overweight is the second leading cause of preventable death.[9] [10] If you think about that for a second, it's actually quite disturbing as it represents almost one out of every two people.

Of course, let's not forget about diabetes, especially Type II, which is directly tied to obesity and being overweight and has also proven to be preventable through diet and exercise.[11] [12] [13]

But as prevalent as the overweight challenges may be they're all trumped by the number one cause of death - heart disease. According to the CDC, one person dies every 36 seconds in the United States from cardiovascular disease, which adds up to 655,000 each year and accounts for 1 in every 4 deaths. Remarkably, studies show that up to 80% of all heart disease is preventable with proper diet and lifestyle changes.[14] [15]

And if heart diseases weren't bad enough, we also have to deal with cancer, which claims roughly 600,000 people each year. But again, there's a silver lining here as American Cancer Researchers have found roughly half of these cases are preventable with proper diet.[16]

Lastly, if finding the motivation to prevent heart disease, diabetes and cancer doesn't push you to change your diet perhaps knowing that over 90% of all hospitalizations from the virus COVID-19 are attributed to underlying conditions including heart disease, cancer, obesity, and diabetes will.[17]

While these statistics may sound morbidly depressing to most, to me they sound incredibly encouraging for the simple fact that five of the top causes of death are in large part preventable by eating the foods outlined in The Power Diet. (Note: this includes Alzheimer's disease and stroke).

This may sound like a bold claim but stick with me and I'll prove it to you with delicious savory meals tested over a million years of evolution and backed by over 240 scientific studies.

Bottom line: If you simply implement the strategies in this book you too can supercharge your immune system and not only build an inhospitable environment for diseases and viral invaders but enjoy more energy, libido and power, which will enable to do way more and live much longer.

What's Your Story?

Are you overweight, underweight, battling an illness, or just desire to live life at a higher level? While we all have different challenges we all have substances, which drain our power and make us more susceptible to illness and disease.

Shortly, we'll take a deep dive into those substances to replace the power drains with the power boosters but before we do, you'll need to make a commitment to take action, without which new power will remain but an illusion.

Personally, I've experimented with diets and solutions for over 20 years but it wasn't until I reached my mid 30's that I really put my foot down and made a non-negotiable agreement with myself to take action and find out what was really draining my power.

This is really important, perhaps even more important than *The Power Diet* itself because without an ironclad agreement to stay committed to forward progress, you'll more likely melt into a couch with a clicker than boost your power and fly away to an exotic adventure.

Accordingly, once you've identified you personal kryptonite we'll be creating a non-negotiable agreement to eliminate power drains. For now, I suggest making an iron clad, non-negotiable goal to simply complete this book. You can do this by setting aside 30 minutes to an hour each day and scheduling some reading time.

Take action now and schedule this time as it could mean the difference between falling prey to one of those top five death traps or flying away on an exotic adventure.

Diets Vs. Lifestyles

If there is one thing I know for certain about food it's this:

Diets come and go while lifestyles remain!

In my initial attempts to recover my own power I, like so many others, sought out the quick solution that would somehow change everything overnight. During this time I tried numerous diets that had been highly recommended including:

- Ayurveda
- Forks Over Knives
- South Beach
- Pritikin
- The Zone
- Ketogenic
- Paleo
- Primal
- Atkins
- Mediterranean
- Plant Paradox
- Bulletproof
- Fat For Fuel

Some of these diets actually came with indisputable evidence, which gave me noticeable results, while some were extreme, based on pseudoscience and were simply unsustainable.

Some contained strategies based on millions of years of evolution, which created sustainable lifestyle changes and formed the backbone of this book, while others sent me back to the toilet with more gut pain or back to bed with a new virus.

After years of intense study and personal experimentation what I realized was that there is a dichotomy in nutrition that most are unaware of. Specifically, on the one hand there are fundamentals of nutrition that affect all of us while on the other there are some unknown quantities that affect each of us uniquely and require more flexible solutions.

These realizations didn't happen overnight. Instead, they took over 15 years of testing and experimentation to find out what clearly does and does not work. I've now taken these revelations and created a sustainable lifestyle, which has had a profound impact on thousands of people's lives.

Most importantly, this simple, yet unique formula sealed the lining of my gut wall, ended the pain, bloating and discomfort, doubled my energy, boosted my immune system, lifted my libido and it can do the same for you!

Don't Believe Everything You Read

Some of what you will hear in this book may contradict and fly in the face of old traditions and outdated nutritional science. But I assure you, they are tried, tested and proven under scientific conditions and have impacted the lives of millions of people for the better. If you have any lingering doubts by the time you finish I encourage you to investigate the over 200 references that back the validity of this book and its strategies when you get to the end.

Even more importantly, I recommend you do not believe what you read just because it came from some well-known guru or doctor or even a scientific study. Instead, the real proof of success will ultimately come from the results you see and feel by testing out the principles of *The Power Diet* or any diet for that matter.

Be Open to Everything and Attached to Nothing

If you're familiar with my training "The Winner's Mindset" you may remember this last statement as a "Master Mantra," which I use in most of my books and trainings.

Given the state of the world right now, (an unprecedented pandemic and the shutdown of worldwide commerce), it's even more important to open up to new ways of living and let go of our old ways, which have created our present circumstances. And if you think the superbugs and viruses like the Coronavirus are gone, think again.

Viruses and bacteria have been around for billions of years, long before our time and as you'll learn later on from a famous battle between two adversaries (Louis Pasteur and Antoine Béchamp) the most important thing you can do has less to do with wearing a mask and hiding in your basement and more to do with boosting your natural immunity by building your power.

Of course, this relates directly to this book as when it comes time to change something you've been doing your whole life – like eating – you'll need to open up to new ways and let go of your attachments to old ways if you are to be successful.

Fortunately, according to studies, having a mindset that seeks growth and new ways (AKA a growth mindset), will give you a big advantage in successfully implementing *The Power Diet* or any other big change as a long-term lifestyle.[18]

So get excited because this is the point where you get to jump off the bandwagon and separate yourself from the herd by letting let go of your attachments to many of the old outdated ways of the past that have not served the greatest version of you. Right now is a massive opportunity for you to expand your physical and mental power, which will allow you to fully express yourself and live into your potential.

Your Diet Is The Front Line

Whether you're trying to beat a virus, lose weight, gain weight, get rid of cancer, look more attractive or solve an issue like leaky gut, if you don't address your diet it doesn't matter how much you exercise, where you come from or what your genetics are.

We eat every day, multiple times per day and as that old tired rephrase goes "you truly are what you eat." As such, your diet represents the front line of both your defense and offense.

This is absolutely critical and according to Doctors like Phil McGuff, your diet actually accounts for about 80 percent of the health benefits derived from a healthy lifestyle, with the remaining 20 percent coming from exercise.   Says McGuff:

"The standard American diet is highly inflammatory. It produces systemic inflammation of an order that is almost beyond belief. In that state, if you do exercise of any significant stress, you're just adding inflammation on top of the inflammation, and you're actually putting yourself at a bit of a risk. I advise people to get their diet straight and then

exercise. Because I think a highly inflammatory diet, in combination with the acute systemic inflammation that occurs as a part of the exercise stimulus, can actually be a negative thing."

Further advice from Michael Mathews, best selling author of "Bigger Leaner Stronger" adds further credence to this statement by proclaiming:

"Eat wrong, and you will stay fat no matter how much cardio you do. Eat wrong, and you stay skinny and weak no matter how much you struggle with weights. Eat right, however, and you can unlock the maximum potential gains from working out."

If you're not already hip to this, according to multiple studies, excessive inflammation is the leading cause of most major diseases including atherosclerosis, arthritis, psoriasis, gout, asthma, allergies and multiple sclerosis, amongst others.[19][20]

The Power Is In The Food

Fortunately, *The Power Diet* is derived from some of the top nutritionists, doctors and scientists in the world and backed by real scientific studies. The basic premise originates from the famous credo of Hippocrates who lived in ancient Greece almost 2,500 years ago and encourage us to:

"Let food be thy medicine and medicine be thy food"

Traditionally regarded as the father of medicine, Hippocrates' revelations about health are used worldwide to this day by doctors and health professionals and it's no wonder why.

Essentially, if you eat the right foods (power foods) this food will function as powerful medicine to heal just about any ailment you can imagine. And if you eat the wrong foods (power drains) this food will function as powerful poison, which can make you sick and kill you.

Specifically, power foods boost your mental and physical power with super powered microbes, enhanced detoxification and reduced inflammation, while power draining foods increase toxins, set your body on fire and kill off all your good microbes. By adding power foods and removing the power drains you'll be much closer to ditching those doctors and the diseases that plague most of humanity.

And while there are several variables that can boost or drain your power, one key element we'll be focusing on is the power of your microbiome - the collective genomes of microbes (bacteria, bacteriophage, fungi, protozoa and viruses) that live within and on your body. This is crucial since your gut wall houses 70% of the cells that make up your immune system.[21]

As New York Times best-selling author and Medical Director of The UltraWellness Center, Dr. Mark Hyman, says:

"You might not attribute digestive problems with allergies, arthritis, autoimmune diseases (irritable bowel syndrome, acne, chronic fatigue), mood disorders, autism, dementia and cancer. Many diseases seemingly unrelated are actually caused by gut problems. If you want to fix your health, start with your gut. Gut health literally affects your entire body."

Fortunately, *The Power Diet* will show you how to rebuild and balance your microbiome in a flexible and sustainable manner by dividing foods into three simple groups as follows:

Power Drain – These foods are toxic for various reasons and should be eliminated from your diet completely.
Power Limit – The foods can boost your power yet drain it when eaten too frequently or in excessive portions. These foods should be consumed on a limited basis – one to three days per week. If you still have limited power after limiting these for 90 days, eliminate them altogether.
Power Boost – These foods turn on your natural ability to cleanse toxins, kill harmful viruses and bacteria, shed fat, and boost energy, strength. But that's not it, they also have the power to boost libido, Testosterone and HGH (human growth hormone) and should take up a majority of your plate at every meal.

Take Action

Throughout this book, you will consistently see the words **"Take Action."** I'm going to assume that if you're reading this book you are seeking new results in your life, which means you must absolutely take action.

Lack of action is the #1 reason people do not succeed in life and without action, your power will only decrease. Consequently, you'll need to make sure you take some form of action each time you see the following words:

"Take Action"

In *The Power Diet,* this will either be a simple act like writing down a key lesson in your smartphone or repeating a phrase so you remember it. If you can't do these simple acts you may as well just give up right now. Strong words perhaps but I'm not interested in just collecting more readers and selling more books. I'm interested in changing your life, that's what I'm here on earth to do, which means you must take some form of action.

Now hopefully you're on board with the crucial nature of taking action, which means it's time for some action.

Question: From this point on you'll need to ask yourself a critical question when you eat your next meal and every other meal for the rest of your life:

Does This Food Give Me Power Or Take It Away?

By asking yourself this simple question you'll begin to create awareness around the food you eat, which will start the experimentation phase of *The Power Diet*. So right now, go ahead and write this question down somewhere in your kitchen or in your smartphone and repeat it at least 5 times. This is really important since it will begin to activate your RAS (reticular activating system).

If you're not already familiar with the RAS, this is a real part of your brain that automatically focuses in on things that are important to you.

Like a homing device, your RAS brings things to your attention and makes them important. For instance, have you ever bought something like a car or jacket and started noticing others who had the same car or jacket? This is your RAS in action!

It's not that you couldn't see these things before, it's just that your RAS wasn't focused on them.

Similarly, if you begin to focus on the level of energy and power associated with the foods you eat, you'll begin to clearly see and feel what foods boost and drain your power. If you can do this consistently over time, you'll begin to automatically refine your diet to find your own personal sweet spot of optimized power where life becomes much easier and more enjoyable.

And since repetition is the mother of all skill, go ahead and repeat this question to yourself right now and remember to ask yourself after each meal:

Did This Food Give Me Power Or Take It Away?

The Three Pillars Of The Power Diet

I believe eating should be simple without having to think a lot when preparing or ordering food. And while food and nutrition are indeed a complex subject, which could be discussed and argued for eons, there are really three key things you need to remember when you buy your food and when you eat it.

I call these "The Three Pillars," due to the fact that when you combine them they support each other like a triangle, which forms one of the most unbreakable foundations in the universe.

Similarly, when you take action to implement the three pillars of *The Power Diet* you too will have an unbreakable foundation from which to support, grow and sustain all of the activities of your life. The three pillars are as follows:

1) **Quality** - What it's made of and where it comes from

2) **Quantity** - How much you should eat

3) **Frequency** - When you should eat

Pillar 1 – Quality

I could've easily called this "What to eat," but that would've distracted you from the most important aspect of what you eat, which is what it's made of and where it comes from. This is by far the largest and most involved of the three pillars so we'll spend a good chunk our time here understanding what "Quality Food" is.

If for instance, you eat non-organic fruits and vegetables grown in the United States, you are more than likely eating low quality food since it's probably laced with glyphosate, a toxic substance found in the pesticide called Round Up, which according to the World Health Organization causes cancer.

And where does glyphosate come from?

Well, that would be Monsanto, one of the most vilified companies on the planet, who has put hundreds of small farmers out of business and acquired hundreds of lawsuits in the process.

Many of these lawsuits are directly related to the destructive and power-sapping effects of their toxic herbicide, Roundup, one of which resulted in a $2.05 billion judgment.

But don't think for a second that the $2.5 billion award windfall didn't come with a heavy price. Recipients Alva and Albert Pilliod used Monsanto's Roundup spray to keep weeds off their driveway for more than two decades and as a result, contracted Non-Hodgkin's Lymphoma (NHL) a potentially fatal cancer.

Of course, this is just one example of how food chemicals can steal your power and send you to the couch, or worse – the graveyard.

Accordingly, in *The Power Diet,* we'll be focusing on increasing the primary elements of food quality that boost power and eliminating the ones that drain your power.

Toxic Vs. Non-Toxic Food

Toxic food, in general, refers to food that has been altered
from its original state and drained of its life giving power.
This power drain can be created by a host of causes such as
pesticides and herbicides but can be lurking in some of the
most unlikely places.

For example, BPA in plastic is known to cause "Metabolic
Syndrome," a cluster of conditions that occur together,
increasing your risk of heart disease, stroke and type 2
diabetes.[22] Make sure you look for signs that say "BPA
Free" whenever you purchase bottled water or any other
product that uses plastic.

Equally as harmful are chemicals used in cooking such as
Teflon, which up until 2013 used a toxic chemical known as
PFOA, to create non-stick cook wear. Even though this toxic
substance has been banned, when heated over 570°F
(300°C), current Teflon coatings begin to break down,
releasing toxic fumes into the air, which can cause
temporary, flu-like symptoms known as polymer fume
fever.[23]

To sum up the effects of these toxins, let's take a look at
the difference between power draining foods and power
boosting foods.

• **Power Drain:** Anything with pesticides, herbicides, plastics or harmful chemicals.
• **Power Boost:** Organic or locally grown without pesticides, herbicides, plastics or harmful chemicals.

Preservatives

Of course, these are just a few of the many toxic substances
that can drain your power. Preservatives can also ruin the

delicate balance of bacteria in your gut, drain your power and make you sick with inflammation, diabetes, metabolic syndrome, obesity, cancer and other not so fun stuff.[24] [25]

If we simply dial back the time before refrigerators (around two hundred years ago) we find the use of natural preservatives like salt and vinegar as a virtual godsend, which enabled populations to thrive in harsh times by preserving meat and vegetables, which were not available.

Sadly, in the interest of profit, big food corporations created chemicals to add longer shelf life to foods. Many of these "preservatives" are highly toxic and should be avoided if at all possible.

Let's take a look at a list of some of the most toxic preservatives so the next time you buy something in a package you can recognize it and choose a more healthy option.

- ✓ BHA and BHT (butylated hydroxyanisole and butylated hydroxytoluene) found in chewing gum, breakfast cereal, crackers, potato chips, etc.

- ✓ TBHQ (tertiary-butyl hydroquinone) is found in instant noodles, candy, etc.

- ✓ Sodium benzoate is found in soft drinks, juices, pickles and salad dressings, etc.

- ✓ Sodium nitrite and nitrate are found in deli meats, bacon ham, smoked fish and hot dogs.

Let's recap what we know about preservatives.

- **Power Drain:** Anything that contains unnatural preservatives like BHT, BHA, TBHQ, sodium benzoate and sodium nitrite and nitrate.

- **Power Boost:** Foods with safe and natural preservatives like apple cider vinegar, salt, lemon or lime.

Additives and Artificial Sweeteners

Additives and artificial sweeteners are equally (pun intended) damaging when it comes to protecting your microbiome and increasing your power. Again, make sure you read labels and if at all possible, forgo ingesting these substances, which can act like poison and make you sick.

- ✓ Equal, Splenda, Sweet'n Low, Aspartame, etc.

- ✓ Trans Fats, Hydrogenated Oils

- ✓ Artificial flavors

- ✓ Monosodium Glutamate (MSG)

- ✓ Artificial Colors (Dyes)

- ✓ High Fructose Corn Syrup (HFCS)

- ✓ GMOs – Genetically modified organisms are a highly debated topic typically focused on cross-bred vegetables and grains.

  Note: Studies show that most pigs raised in the US who are typically fed a mixture of GE soy and corn causes severe inflammation in the pigs' stomachs. Overall, inflammation levels were found to be 2.6 times higher in GE-fed pigs than those fed a non-GE diet. The GE diet test simulated a typical American, who will be exposed to a variety of different GE foods through his or her daily diet, rather than just one at a time.[26]

**Can you guess the one thing
these foods all have in common?**

If you guessed that they create more inflammation, which leads to more disease, you are correct! Since eliminating

these power drains is so important, let's go ahead and recap
what we know about additives and artificial sweeteners.

* **Power Drain:** Any food with artificial additives,
  hydrogenated oils, fake sweeteners or GMOs.

* **Power Boost:** Foods with a very low amount of
  natural sweeteners like honey or stevia.

***Note:** all sweets are highly addictive and can lead to
inflammatory conditions. Make sure to moderate sweets,
including the natural ones.

Fried And Grilled Foods

If you're looking at the title of this next section and find
yourself scratching your head or mumbling "no way, not my
grilled meat, not my French fries," take a deep breath and
relax.

First off, if you follow The Power Diet and practice it daily
you'll eventually get to the point where your newly enhanced
detoxification system can handle an occasional outing at the
local burger joint which features an overcooked
cheeseburger with a plate of fries dipped in ranch dressing.

Secondly, by shedding some light on the darkness of toxic
food and all the pain it creates, your newly enhanced
knowledge and motivation will more than likely steer you
clear of these power drains and instead set you free to build
superhuman power.

Speaking of which, here's a not so fun fact: Fried foods,
which are often cooked in vegetable oil, have been linked to
inflammatory diseases like cancer, diabetes, heart disease,
and obesity.[27]

Not so fun fact #2: French fries contain trans fats which
can lead to colon cancer and when cooked at high
temperatures can create acrylamides, which are known

neurotoxins found in paint thinner and have been shown to kill animals.[28] [29]

If not eating French fries anymore worries you, it's important to understand that your body craves the fat and carbohydrates contained in those fries, so you're not completely wrong for eating them.

Unfortunately, as evidenced by these and many other studies, the type of carbs and fats contained in French fries drain your power.

Essentially, while you may love fried or grilled foods, they may not love you back the way you think they do.

For example, according to multiple studies, when proteins are heated to the point that the flesh starts to brown and blacken, heterocyclic amines (HCAs) begin to form, some of which are known carcinogens. Diets with high exposures to HCAs are correlated with higher rates of cancers of the pancreas, colon and digestive tract.[30] [31]

If you're a grilled food lover, this might not be the best news you've ever heard (right now) but there are a few workarounds.

For example, by marinating with acidic ingredients like lemon, lime or vinegar (not sugar) you can significantly reduce HCA levels. And to ensure against any further power draining effects of grilling, make sure your marinade includes high potency antioxidant herbs like basil, mint, rosemary, oregano, or marjoram or just add them on top with some oil.

Let's recap what we know about fried and grilled foods.

<table>
<tr><td>

- **Power Drain:** Anything fried and most grilled food including French fries, fish sticks, onion rings, donuts, grilled meats and blackened foods.

</td></tr>
<tr><td>

- Power Limit – Lightly grilled meats with protective marinades, herbs and spices.

</td></tr>
<tr><td>

- Power Boost: Fresh whole foods and protein sources that have not been fried grilled or overly cooked.

</td></tr>
</table>

Whole Foods Vs. Highly Refined Foods

On The Power Diet, you'll gain the most power from foods that have not been altered much from their original state and are considered whole foods.

In contrast, low-quality foods that create a power deficit tend to be overly processed and high in refined sugar. According to studies, highly refined foods can increase the production of inflammatory markers and lead to diabetes, hypertension and cardiovascular disease.[32]

Let's take a look at the difference between the power drains and power boosters.

> - **Power Drain:** Alcohol, Coca Cola, candy, white sugar, pastries, donuts, pizza, apple juice, etc.
>
> - **Power Boost:** Foods that have not been altered or processed from their original states like blueberries, broccoli, carrots, cauliflower, walnuts, almonds, sweet potatoes and other power foods.

Coke And Pizza – Nick Jonas Case Study

You may have noticed two of the world's most favorite foods Coke and Pizza on that power drain list but what you may not have noticed is the staggering amount of studies that have shown how refined carbohydrates like pizza and coca cola can lead to diabetes, hypertension and cardiovascular disease. [33] [34] [35]

As a musician, I often watch documentaries on rock bands in the hopes of learning something new. In "Chasing Happiness," the three Jonas Brothers document their meteoric rise to fame and the inevitable trials that created their eventual demise as a band.

One of the most notable of these trials was the addiction, not to drugs (like most other rock stars), but to pizza and Coke by the youngest of the three brothers Nick Jonas. Apparently, Nick was scarfing down pizza and Coke regularly, which depleted his power until diabetes sidelined him to the hospital and threatened to end his life and career.

Of course, Nick isn't alone in this dilemma as the pizza and soda industry sell billions of dollars worth of their life draining products each year to millions of unsuspecting customers.

And while cauliflower pizza may not sound so appetizing to you right now, once you create a new habit of eating power producing foods, you'll more than likely be addicted to feeling good and won't crave these power drains.

Recap Of Power Draining Toxins

Clearly, there are many ways to toxify and drain power from food. Remembering these can make all the difference in creating a day filled with energy, smiles and productivity or a month in bed with a flu virus or a trip to the hospital for a shot of insulin. So let's go ahead and bolster our defenses by recapping what we know so far about the Power Drains.

We now know that food that has been altered from its original state can drain your power if it contains the following substances:

- ✓ Toxic herbicides and pesticides

- ✓ Unnatural Preservatives & Additives

- ✓ GMOs

- ✓ Artificial Sweeteners

- ✓ Fried food, grilled or blackened food

- ✓ Hydrogenated oils (trans fats)

✓   Over processed and refined foods

Take Action – Eliminate Toxins

To make sure you're not poisoning yourself with poor quality food and draining your power there are two key actions you'll need to take as follows:

1) **Limit if not eliminate packaged, canned and processed foods.** As you'll soon discover in our raw vs. cooked food section, with some rare exceptions, these foods are close to dead (devoid of any significant life). This is where you'll find 90% of the low quality food.

2) **Start Reading Labels** - If for some reason you do buy something that was modified or processed from its original state you'll need to get in the habit of reading labels. If it doesn't have a label make sure you ask the vendor the following question:

What's In It?

If you find ingredients you can't pronounce, chances are it's toxic and more than likely made in a lab instead of a garden. And if you find any of the above mentioned power drains in front of you simply pass and find something else that hasn't been toxified from its original state.

Once you find your power restored and your mind firing on all cylinders you'll have created an environment where no illness or cancer can live. And… I guarantee you'll be glad you took action.

Antinutrients Kill Your Power

Ok so let's say you've gotten rid of the toxic power drains mentioned above and you're eating whole foods but you still struggle with inflammation, weight gain, digestive issues, arthritis, cardiovascular issues, low libido or just low energy.

If any of this sounds familiar, you may be struggling with antinutrients, plant compounds that reduce your body's ability to absorb essential nutrients and wreak havoc on your microbiome.

And just when you thought it was safe to dive into the garden of plant based eating because documentaries like "Game Changers" punched a hole in the meatball manifesto of America, along comes the discovery of antinutrients (massive power drains) found primarily in plants.

But again, don't worry, because we'll be navigating around these pitfalls with some brilliant strategies that optimize plant power while at the same time minimizing the power drains.

First off, it's important to understand that antinutrients, in large part, are built-in defense mechanisms, which function to perpetuate the species of each plant. Some of these are so toxic they can literally kill you.[36]

In fact, castor beans contain an antinutrient called "lectins," which contains ricin, a lethal substance used as a poison during the cold war.

In 2018 ricin was detected in mail sent to The Pentagon and addressed to Secretary of Defense Jim Mattis and President Donald Trump (among others). Had they inhaled the ricin they would've most likely died in few days or less.

But this is just one way a plant protects itself. As you can imagine, there are many ways they do this, which is another in-depth subject of which several great books have been written including, "The Blood Type Diet" by Dr. Peter J D'Adamo and "The Plant Paradox" by Dr. Steven Gundry.

But again, our goal is to uncover the root solution and not get bogged down in all the details, so let's take a look at what science says about some of the biggest antinutrient culprits and how we can eliminate their potential to drain your power.

Tannins

First on the list of antinutrients are tannins, a class of antioxidant polyphenols that may impair the digestion of various nutrients, in particular, iron.[37]

While tannins can be found in various plants, they are most common in coffee and tea and can bind with iron present in plant-based foods, rendering it unavailable for absorption.[38]

While research indicates that this effect is not likely to cause significant harm in people with healthy iron levels, if you have an iron deficiency it could cause anemia and some other not so fun diseases.[39] [40]

How can I limit this power drain of tannins?

Personally, when I wake up in the morning after I've had my alkaline water, I drink a variety of green teas like matcha, yerba mate and once in a while, coffee. What I noticed was that each time I drank any of these from a low-grade source I felt nauseous. Later on, I found out this was one of the side effects of too much tannin and when I switched to a higher-grade organic brand I didn't have this problem. [41]

As for the compromised iron absorption, just make sure you drink your tea between meals so the tannins don't bind to the iron in your food (assuming there's iron in your food). And if you feel nauseous make sure you dump that tea or coffee in the trash and buy an organic high-grade source instead.

Lastly, it's important to limit your consumption of these beverages as too many tannins can not only disrupt the absorption of key nutrients but overconsumption of caffeine can jack up your cortisol, put you in fight or flight mode and create all kinds of power drains like anxiety,[42] insulin insensitivity,[43] insomnia,[44] digestive issues,[45] muscle breakdown,[46] addiction,[47] high blood pressure,[48] and fatigue.[49]

Yep, that's right, instead of a boost, too much caffeine will eventually drain you, create fatigue and lead to adrenal burnout.

If you feel the need for constant caffeine, you're either addicted, lacking in sleep, metabolic inflexibility or a combination of these. If this seems like a challenge for you, dial it down by sticking to 1 cup of caffeinated beverages per day maximum and instead of relying on caffeine for your energy, make sure you stick to The Power Diet foods, which will balance your hormones and bring you back your natural internal power.

Limit caffeinated beverages to 1 per day!

Oxalates

Oxalates are organic compounds found in leafy greens like spinach, beets, kale and Swiss chard, which can bind to minerals like calcium and inhibit absorption as well as create kidney stones.[50] [51]

If you've ever had a kidney stone you know this is a serious problem and if you haven't all you need to know is this: The pain from a kidney stone can be equated to the pain a female goes through when giving birth. Believe me, it's no fun, I've been there and you want nothing to do with it.

Unless you're eating a 100% animal based diet you will be ingesting some oxalates so instead of trying to get rid of all oxalates, our goal here is to simply limit them. To do this we'll only eat them raw on occasion and for the most part, we'll steam, boil, lightly sauté or pressure-cook them, which can eliminate up to 87% of the oxalates.[52]

Lastly, you also want to make sure you're drinking ample alkaline fluids throughout the day as lack of hydration has also been linked to Kidney Stones.[53] (See The Power Diet Master Guide for recommendations).

Steam, boil, lightly sauté or pressure cook high oxalate veggies and limit eating them raw!

Protease Inhibitors

Protease inhibitors are found in a variety of plants especially seeds, grains, and legumes and can disrupt the digestion of protein by inhibiting digestive enzymes.

While some studies have found that soaking legumes like peas for 6-18 hours decreased lectins by 38-50%, tannins by 13-25% and protease inhibitors by 28-30%,[54] this effect is much less pronounced in other legumes like kidney beans, Soybeans, and fava beans.[55]

Phytates & Phytic Acid

Similar to protease inhibitors, phytate is also found primarily in seeds, grains, and legumes and can reduce the absorption of minerals like iron, zinc, magnesium, and calcium.[56]

One of the major challenges of soy-based products is their high level of phytic acid. Fortunately, fermented soy (AKA tempeh), removes most of the harmful phytic acid. In fact, studies show sprouting can reduce phytate by 37-81% in various types of grains and legumes and by combining this with fermentation both phytate and lectins can be significantly degraded. [57] [58] [59] [60]

Lectins

Lectins are found in all plants and can react negatively with the human microbiome especially when it comes to seeds, legumes, and grains. Similar to our other antinutrients, reactive lectins can also disrupt the absorption of nutrients and wreak havoc on your microbiome.[61] [62]

Before we move on, let's pause for a second and ponder the common pattern created by antinutrients and what this means for your daily diet.

With the exception of our first two power drains (tannins and oxalates), the last three all come in the form of seeds, grains and legumes.

The overwhelming data that seeds, grains and legumes can wreck your gut by creating inflammation at this point is simply indisputable. And to demonstrate the power draining effects let me share one of many personal experiences with one of my favorite food combinations.

Peanut Butter And Chocolate

There really aren't a whole lot of things on this planet that satisfy the pallet so immensely than combining rich chocolate with creamy peanut butter. Sadly, every single time I eat peanut butter, within about 12-24 hours my knuckles in my hands start to swell up and I feel like an arthritic 90 year old man.

While I've intuitively known peanuts to be a problem for years, my wishful thinking recently guided me to experiment with peanut butter in the hopes that somehow, after not eating peanut butter for several years, my body would now tolerate it.

After indulging in roughly two tablespoons of organic high-grade peanut butter, sure enough, within 24-48 hours I could barely close my fists from the intense inflammation. But after a week of not eating peanut butter, the inflammation in my hands completely went away.

Since I had eaten the same thing every day for the last two months I had indisputable evidence that peanut butter was indeed the trigger.

If this is at all disheartening, have heart peanut lovers, because I'm going to turn you on to another nut that tastes just like it - minus the problematic lectins.

Keep in mind, for some people, not only will peanuts create autoimmune disorders but other nuts can have the same effect. We'll talk more about those later on.

And while you may not be as sensitive to foods as I am and you may not shrivel up with arthritis from peanuts there is a good chance your power is being drained from reactive lectins on a daily basis whether you're aware of it or not.

So right now I'd like to ask you to again put aside your inner critic and consider how the not so obvious may be sucking away years of your life and more importantly, how you could potentially progress by leaps and bounds by simply taking a few key power drains out of your diet.

But first, just what are these strange plant substances called lectins?

What Are Lectins?

Lectins are also antinutrients, which are a type of toxic protein substance found in all plants. Similar to our other antinutrients, lectins are built in defenses to deter animals (including humans) from eating plants so they can perpetuate their species.

While some lectins are dangerous, some are perfectly suitable if not beneficial for the human microbiome. For example, some lectins can act as antioxidants, which protect cells from damage caused by free radicals. They can also slow down digestion and the absorption of carbohydrates, which may prevent sharp rises in blood sugar and high insulin levels.

In contrast, studies suggest that roughly 30% of the harmful lectins in the modern diet can reduce the body's ability to absorb nutrients and eating large amounts of them can damage your gut wall. This causes irritation that can result in symptoms like diarrhea and vomiting and can also prevent your gut from absorbing nutrients properly.[63]

This, of course, is highly significant since your gut wall contains 70% of your immune power and once this is compromised all hell breaks loose.

For example, imagine that your ideal gut looks like a tropical rainforest, with lots of species working in harmony to support and protect a lush and balanced ecosystem.

Similarly, your gut is supported and protected by trillions of microorganisms (also called microbiota or microbes) of thousands of different species.[64] These not only include bacteria but fungi, parasites, and viruses. Yes, that's right, viruses!

In a healthy person, these "bugs" coexist peacefully, with the largest numbers found in the small and large intestines as well as throughout your entire body.

Unfortunately, once you introduce certain reactive lectins they breach your gut wall and start to burn down your forest.

Quite ironically, if you've heard of the "Carnivore Diet" or the "Paleo" diet where people have been able to cure themselves of autoimmune disorders like arthritis, or leaky gut syndrome there's a good chance that most of the benefits of these diets are coming from the fact that they've eliminated forest-burning lectins like grains and beans.

Adding fuel to the forest fire are all those toxins in your food we talked about earlier, which makes you acidic and create the perfect environment for power draining invaders to take residence in your gut. Oh yeah, and did I mention that they also eat your food and take a crap that your body has to somehow clean up and process?

But that's not it. You must also consider all the antibiotics you've taken over the last 10-15 years which have carpet bombed your forest indiscriminately, killing off both good and bad bacteria, as well as the NSAID'S (Ibuprofen, Advil, Naproxen, etc.), which have been scientifically proven to blow holes in the lining of your gut wall.[65]

Now considering all the warfare and forest fires already happening in your microbiome, can you imagine what happens by adding harmful lectins on top of all that? Its no wonder the antacid industry is selling so much product. As best selling author Dr. Steven Gundry says:

"In the gut, lectins flip a switch that creates a space between intestinal cells, allowing bacteria and lipopolysaccharides (LPS) to cross the gut wall," he explains. Once these things breach the gut wall, they can enter the bloodstream and potentially trigger bad reactions throughout the body."

Sadly, this breach kills off most of your good bacteria and leaves your forest unprotected, at which point more invaders and gang members like pathogens, viruses, fungi and parasites take over and pillage your forest of its power.

Perhaps most surprisingly, the highest concentrations of antinutrients are found in supposedly healthy foods like legumes, grains, and nightshade vegetables.

Although there are ways to reduce harmful lectin content by cooking, sprouting, or fermenting, some foods like wheat should be avoided altogether. And while this may be upsetting for many, the research and evidence clearly indicate that some of the most troublesome lectins like wheat germ agglutinin (WGA) interferes with gene expression, increases inflammation and disrupts your endocrine function.[66]

According to Dr. Amy Myers, lectins are also problematic in GMO foods since these foods are engineered with more insecticides to deter insects from eating them. And while this strategy may yield more crops, essentially, by eating GMO foods you're most likely getting more antinutrients and with it more inflammation and the diseases that are triggered.[67]

And perhaps the final blow to eating wheat is the fact that when you eat it you're ingesting reactive lectin proteins called amylase-trypsin inhibitors (ATIs), which can trigger inflammation related to chronic diseases such as multiple sclerosis, asthma and rheumatoid arthritis.[68]

As you can see, antinutrients like lectins found in seeds, grains and legumes can drain your power and it's very difficult to remove all lectins no matter how many ways you prepare them. This is critical so I'm going to say something you definitely need to pay attention to:

Most Antinutrients Are Found In Seeds, Grains And Legumes – Either Limit or Eliminate Them

Again, if this worries you, take a deep breath and relax; there are plenty of great options we'll be revealing shortly that taste even better than wheat and you can use a combination of soaking, sprouting, fermenting and pressure-cooking to remove many antinutrients in seeds and legumes.

We'll talk about those foods shortly, for now, if you have any doubts about the realities of antinutrients I highly recommend you take a deeper dive into the subject as there is plenty of science out there. If you do, you will find thousands upon thousands of case studies from people who have cured ailments including obesity, leaky gut syndrome, arthritis, psoriasis, Crohn's disease, heart disease and many others by removing harmful antinutrients from their diet.

At this point, you're probably wondering just what are the foods with antinutrients. So let's break it down into our three categories.

Power Drain: Any foods, which are high in antinutrients that interfere with your body's natural function should be limited or removed completely. This may differ from person to person so make sure you take into consideration the recommended action. Below are the main power drains, take a mental note if you have a lot of these in your diet.

- ✓ Legumes - Red kidney beans, peas, soybean products and lentils (see exceptions below).

- ✓ Nuts & Seeds - Pumpkin, chia seeds, sunflower, peanuts, cashews

    Special Note: If you have a clearly negative response (inflammation, rashes or seizures) from other nuts and seeds like pistachios you may have extra sensitivity. In this case, you should remove them for 30 days then retest to see if they affect you negatively again. If they do eliminate them.

- ✓ Grains – Whole wheat, amaranth, buckwheat, barley, corn, quinoa, oats, Kamut, (see exceptions below).

- ✓ Vegetables – Eggplant, potatoes, tomatoes, peppers, zucchini and cucumbers (For exceptions see additional preparation below).

- ✓ Fruits – All high sugar fruits and fruits not in season

- ✓ Dairy – Milk, yogurt and cheese with casein A1 (especially those derived from grain or soy fed animals)

- ✓ Meats, Poultry & Fish Fed Corn & Soy

    Note: Similar to the GMO pig food example, when it comes to animal and fish products you must also take into consideration what that creature ate. Whatever they ate, if you eat them, you'll be eating the same thing. Conventionally processed dairy, meat, poultry and fish fed with GMO corn and soy is loaded with reactive lectins that could be draining your power every day – eliminate it!

✓ Oils – Soy, grapeseed, corn, peanut, cottonseed, safflower, sunflower, partially hydrogenated vegetable or canola (AKA trans fats).

Power Limit: Since many lectins and polyphenols are actually beneficial, the goal of *The Power Diet* is not to eliminate them but simply limit them. The following are foods that can be beneficial in limited quantities.

✓ Legumes, lentils and beans, which have been soaked, sprouted, and pressure-cooked

✓ Quinoa and potatoes (new, brown, red), which have been pressure-cooked (soaking in water and sprouting prior to pressure cooking can help eliminate even more lectins).

✓ Green tea or coffee with tannins should not exceed 1-2 cups per day

✓ Raw beets, kale, chard, collards and spinach with high oxalate content

✓ Peeled and deseeded tomatoes, cucumber, pumpkin, peppers, zucchini and squash.

✓ Cooked shallots and mushrooms

✓ White rice, millet, fermented sourdough, resistant starch powder.

✓ Dairy - Type 2 casein dairy products do not contain reactive lectins like Type 1 casein. Look for "Type 2" "Grass Fed" at your local grocer or choose goat or sheep dairy, which doesn't have Type 1 or 2.

✓ Meat and Poultry – Choose organic, grass fed and
pasture raised.

Since eliminating certain foods with problematic antinutrients
like legumes and grains from your diet can be a major shock
to most, I'll offer some workarounds for those that want to
include a limited quantity of these in their diet.

While it's virtually impossible to eliminate all harmful
lectins, you can prepare or buy some of these foods
fermented, sprouted, soaked and pressure-cooked. We
already talked about this briefly but it's worth taking another
look to cast a little more light on some of the details.

Boosting Fruits, Veggies, Nuts & Seeds

- **Get Rid of the Skin & Seeds** - The skin (or hull) and
  seeds of fruits, nuts, seeds and vegetables tend to
  contain the highest amounts of antinutrients. For
  example, seeds and skins from peppers and tomatoes
  contain lectins and tannins that can cause indigestion
  and leaky gut but if you remove them by blanching the
  skin and cutting out the seeds you can avoid most of the
  toxic lectins.   A good example would be tomato paste or
  tomato sauce, which doesn't have skins or seeds.
  Almond skins can also be problematic. Try buying
  blanched almonds or blanching them yourself.

- **Eat Fermented Veggies** – Fermentation creates healthy
  bacteria that reduce harmful antinutrients in vegetables
  while at the same time rebuilds your forest and can be
  eaten daily in staples like kimchi, sauerkraut, cucumbers,
  carrots, and other veggies.

Boosting Grains

- **Get Rid Of The Hull** - According to Dr. Steven Gundry,
  the hull of the rice grain contains all the dangerous
  lectins, which means you should avoid brown rice. So

while white rice (preferably jasmine) may not have much nutritional content, this carb heavy food can be eaten in limited quantities.

- **Fermented Bread** - Fermentation also reduces harmful lectins in the hull of wheat when baking sourdough bread, which effectively breaks down most of the gluten and other harmful lectins. Just make sure you eat fermented sourdough in moderation as it does not have much nutrition and can eventually drain your power.

Boosting Beans, Grains & Seeds

- **Sprouting** – By sprouting or buying sprouted beans, grains and seeds you can deactivate some but not all lectins and there are exceptions. For example, by sprouting alfalfa legumes the lectin content is actually enhanced. Nuts, seeds and grains seem to benefit most from sprouting.

- **Use a Pressure Cooker** – By using a pressure cooker or buying pressure-cooked foods you can neutralize many antinutrients from foods like beans, legumes, tomatoes, potatoes and quinoa. You can also buy organic BPA free canned beans from Eden Foods, which have been soaked, sprouted and pressure-cooked (check www.ChadScottCoaching.com/resources for more recommendations). Just keep in mind, there are exceptions, where pressure cooking alone can not remove lectins. This includes: wheat, oats, rye, barley and spelt. Again, if you're a grain lover, don't worry, we'll talk about some tasty replacements shortly, which will help you restore full power. **Note:** Slow cookers, which cook at low temperatures, are insufficient to remove most lectins.

If you do not see a power surge after 3 months on *The Power Diet,* try eliminating all "Power Limiting" foods as well as all "Power Draining" foods.

Power Boost: The power boosters include whole foods that do not have high levels of antinutrients, which your body readily absorbs and assimilates without any adverse effects. This includes:

- ✓ Nuts – almonds (blanched), walnuts, pecans, pistachios, macadamia, pine, brazil, chestnut

- ✓ Seeds – Sesame, hemp, flax

- ✓ Vegetables – Avocado, broccoli, asparagus and cauliflower. Romaine, butter leaf and red leaf lettuces. Olives, celery and bok choy. Cooked kale, chard, collards, beets, spinach and Brussels sprouts. Parsley, cilantro, fennel, jicama, onions, leeks, frisee, cabbage, dandelion greens, radishes, artichoke, endive, radicchio and arugula.

- ✓ Tubers – Carrots, sweet potatoes, yams (these are exceptions to the nightshades and do not have overly reactive lectins).

- ✓ Fruits – coconut, low sugar fruits like apples, pears, apricots and berries when in season

- ✓ Fermented Foods - kimchi, sauerkraut, coconut yogurt and apple cider vinegar.

- ✓ Fish - Choose wild caught low mercury versions including sardines, sockeye salmon, anchovies, mackerel, cod haddock and petrale sole.

- ✓ Oils – Olive, coconut, macadamia, MCT, avocado, perilla, walnut, red palm, rice bran, sesame, cod.

Take Action – Limit or Eliminate Antinutrients

Once you've gotten clear on what foods you need to limit and eliminate, the quickest way to boost your power is to start eliminating the other Power Draining Foods for at least 30 days then retest your power.

Removing problematic foods one at a time is crucial! If you've been eating a lot of these your whole life it could be quite challenging to suddenly stop eating them all at once.

For example, if you love eating whole grain cereal for breakfast then a sandwich with tomatoes, pasteurized cheese, packaged meat and whole wheat bread for lunch, it could be challenging to eliminate all of these at once.

While you can indeed eliminate and replace them with some of the power boosting options, if this seems like an overwhelming task you can start by just eliminating all the grains with lectins that have been shown to create inflammation and simply can't be removed with preparation.

Specifically, I recommend removing wheat, brown rice, corn, oats, rye, barley and spelt. Occasionally, you can eat fermented sourdough bread or white rice, which have had most of their power draining lectins removed. Just keep in mind, these are high in carbohydrates, which as you'll soon learn can drain your power as well; so make sure you limit them.

To avoid the power drain from these grains, your new goal on *The Power Diet* will be to replace these "Power Drains" with power boosting starches like yams, sweet potatoes, carrots and other tubers as well as grain alternatives like cassava, coconut and almond.

We'll talk specifics on recipes and exactly what will be in your daily Power Meals later, for now, it's important to take action by removing these power drain grains for at least 30 days and notice if you feel a power boost with more sustained energy throughout the day.

If you're working out (hopefully with my *Fired Up* program) you should also notice more power, stronger workouts and better sleep. And make sure you check your libido. If you've been diligent in removing the power draining foods, you'll most likely feel more sexually potent.

Next, once you've removed those toxic grain drains, go ahead and remove your proteins from the "Power Drain" lists above. Just follow the recommendations for another 30 days then assess your overall power again and ask yourself that all-important question we listed earlier:

Did This Food Give Me Power Or Take It Away?

Continue doing this 30-day cycle of ditching "Power Draining Foods" until you've ditched them all.

Eventually, what you'll most likely notice is a craving or temptation to go back to some of those Power Draining Foods. This isn't something to be avoided. In fact, I recommend retesting yourself with some of the Power Draining Foods to confirm they really are draining your power and wreaking havoc on your mind, body and quality of life. This pain should be a powerful reminder not to eat them again.

Keep in mind, this cycling phase may take more than 30 days, so be patient and remember… it took months, if not years, to get to where you are now. To change all that history of toxification and sugar burning may simply take more time, so just keep going and give yourself a good 3-6 months to fully feel the effects of lifestyle changes.

**Eliminate at least 1-3 power draining foods
every 30 days!**

Over Cooking Kills Power

While eating raw vs. cooked food has been a heated debate for years, the simple fact is, when you cook most of your food you lose more than you gain.

Yes, certain vegetables like broccoli and carrots can be difficult to digest in their raw state and can give you more of certain nutrients by lightly steaming or sautéing them but the sad fact is, our culture has been conditioned to fear raw food.

Since truth is a potent destroyer of fear, let's take a quick journey into history when all this paranoia of eating raw food began.

If we dial back the timeline to the 18th Century we find an infamous battle between two well-known scientists Louis Pasteur (1822-1895) and Antoine Béchamp (1816-1908).

While both of these men wanted to make an impact on the world with their work, they eventually became adversaries with two strikingly different opinions about where disease comes from. Just check out this chart below:

GERM THEORY (PASTEUR)	CELLULAR THEORY (BÉCHAMP)
1. The body is sterile.	Microbes exist naturally in the body.
2. Disease arises from micro-organisms outside the body.	Disease arises from micro-organisms within the cells of the body.
3. Micro-organisms are generally to be guarded against.	These intracellular micro-organisms normally function to build and assist in the metabolic processes of the body.
4. The function of micro-organisms is constant.	The function of these organisms changes to assist in the catabolic processes of the host organism when that organism dies or is injured, which may be chemical as well as mechanical.
5. The shapes and colours of micro-organisms are constant.	Micro-organisms are pleomorphic (having many forms): they change their shapes and colors (shape-shift) to reflect the condition of the host.
6. Every disease is associated with a particular microorganism.	Every disease is associated with a particular condition.
7. Micro-organisms are primary causal agents.	Disease results when microbes change form, function, and toxicity according to the terrain of the host.
8. Disease can "strike" anybody.	Disease is built by unhealthy conditions.
9. To prevent disease we have to "build defences."	To prevent disease we have to create health.

Turns out just about everything old Louis proposed created inflammation and has, for the most part, been debunked. Quite ironically, Mr. Pasteur, for which pasteurization was named, suffered from two strokes, ate a lot of power draining food and died a lot earlier than Antoine.

Unfortunately, over 100 years later we're still eating predominantly pasteurized foods (at least in the United States) that have been cooked to 161 degrees, which has created loads of inflammation and disease, the evidence of which you'll soon learn, is overwhelming.

Of course, Hippocrates, the father of medicine himself discovered long ago that the real challenge was not the invaders from the outside but the power of the host to fight off invaders from both the inside and outside as he also so famously declared:

"It is more important to know what sort of person has a disease than to know what sort of disease a person has."

For instance, if we took two people, one who ate fast food or just too much food and rarely exercised and one ate power foods and exercised regularly and exposed them both to the Coronavirus, can you guess who more likely be hospitalized and die?

Since a poor diet and lack of exercise are known contributors to heart disease, obesity, diabetes and a host of other ailments we'd be wise to bet on the first person and for several good reasons.[69]

This relates directly to Hippocrates's famous declaration and that study we mentioned earlier from the CDC where researchers found the majority of hospitalized patients due to COVID-19 had preexisting conditions. Specifically, about 90% of patients had one or more underlying conditions the most common of which were hypertension (49.7%), obesity (48.3%), chronic lung disease (34.6%), diabetes mellitus (28.3%), and cardiovascular disease (27.8%).[70]

My own cousin is married to a super healthy guy who contracted the Coronavirus and unknowingly gave it to his family. Since he ate mostly power foods and exercised regularly he showed no signs of the virus while his family, who did not eat many power foods or exercise regularly, got really ill.

With all this mounting evidence, it's time to return to Béchamp's cellular theory, stop making excuses for our poor health and start looking within. And who better to put the cherry on top than our father of medicine Hippocrates who said:

"Natural forces within us are the true healers of disease"

So why did everyone believe old Louis and start pasteurizing food by cooking out most of the good stuff, while old Antoine got lost in the shuffle?

Apparently, old Louis was a good con artist. In a 250-page thesis on Antoine Béchamp, Marie Nonclercq, doctor of pharmacy, explains the clear advantage that Pasteur had over Béchamp:

"He was a falsifier of experiments and their results, where he wanted the outcomes to be favorable to his initial ideas."

Ok so maybe we've been duped into believing some false evidence appearing real (FEAR) but don't worry. If you're thinking you may need to give up cooking, just remember, this is not an extreme diet.

To be clear, *The Power Diet* is NOT a completely raw diet. As just mentioned, there are some foods, which release more power steamed or boiled than if they were eaten raw.

For example, carrots steamed or boiled release more carotenoids important for visual function than if they were eaten raw. [71] In the same token we must also acknowledge the fact that when you cook anything you also lose something and in the case of carrots and cruciferous veggies you lose vitamin C content.

But let's say you have challenges digesting raw carrots, broccoli or zucchini and decide to cook them and supplement with vitamin C to replace any of the negative aspects of cooking. In this case, the method you use to cook also makes a big difference.

In a report published in the Journal of Agriculture and Food Chemistry, researchers demonstrated how boiling and steaming better preserves antioxidants, particularly carotenoid, in carrots, zucchini and broccoli, than frying.[72]

While this all may seem like a lot to digest (pun intended), you don't need to completely eliminate cooked foods. Instead, similar to our lectin draining foods we'll simply limit them and the level of heat used to cook them in order to boost overall power.

The Guru Trap

If we look into the general mindset of a typical American, one of the biggest problems of cooked and pasteurized foods is how most people easily fall prey to "The Guru Trap."

In other words, they believe Doctors and Scientists (remember Louis Pasture) simply because they have an advanced degree or plaque on their wall that says they completed school.

Unfortunately, guys like Pasteur were educated and trained to treat the effects of pathogens by eliminating them with drugs and surgery instead of looking for the root or cause of the problem.

This may be helpful when someone tears off their arm in a car accident or has a cancerous tumor that needs to be removed. But for the majority of cases, when requires medical attention, treating the effects simply does not solve the root of the problem and as a consequence, the problem just keeps returning.

In reality, most MD's have very limited knowledge of nutrition. I know at least a half a dozen personally who have eaten mostly cooked foods their whole lives and either suffered from a heart attack or died from cancer or stroke (remember Dr. Atkins?).

Fortunately, we're about to cast some bright sunshine on the darkness of dead food and boost your power to the heights of the Himalayas (pink salt anybody?).

The 3 Main Power Drains Associated With Cooking Food

If you've ever felt tired after eating or just sluggish in general this next section may open your eyes to a new approach in gaining more energy. Basically, there are three main challenges with cooking food, which science has proven in multiple studies to drain your power.

1) **Enzymes are De-stabilized** – Too much cooked food can make you feel slow and sluggish since in many cases digestion and assimilation are compromised.[73]

2) **Acidity Increases and Alkalinity Decreases** – Food cooked over 118 degrees changes the chemical composition and the pH level, which can make you sluggish and create more inflammation, arthritis, cancer, stroke, dementia, and other not so fun stuff.[74]

3) **Megahertz Energy & Nutrients are Lost** – Think less power here! Literally, by eating too much cooked food you won't be able to think as quickly or clearly since neurotransmitter messengers can be compromised, cells depleted and power diminished.[75]

Enzymes – Your Army Of Helpers

First off, let's talk about enzymes, which are critical as they break stuff down and clean stuff up. Without them, you can't digest and assimilate life-giving nutrients, foods start to stagnate, putrefy and eventually you become toxic and sick.

Essentially, there are two main enzyme classifications, endogenous, which are produced by your pancreas and other cells, and exogenous, which are produced outside your body mostly by raw foods.

Right now we're talking about exogenous enzymes in food, which according to studies can become de-stabilized at temperatures as low as 72 degrees.[76]

Considering the fact that most cooked foods are heated way beyond 72 degrees (pasteurized milk is heated to between 145 - 300 degrees Fahrenheit), when it comes to preserving enzymes this is obviously not a good thing.

Dr. Humbart Santillo, a Naturopathic doctor, provides an excellent explanation of how exogenous enzymes are used to break down food into smaller and more operable nutritional units as follows:

"The more one gets of the exogenous enzymes, the less will have to be borrowed [from the body.] One can live many years on a cooked food diet, but eventually, this will cause cellular enzyme exhaustion, which lays the foundation for a weak immune system and ultimately—disease."

I don't know about you but that doesn't exactly sound like a power building strategy to me. And this is just one point of view from a mounting stockpile of evidence, which clearly demonstrates that eating too much cooked food is making us sick.

In another study performed at the University of California, researchers measured the digestion of bread that had been cooked three ways: mildly, normally and over-baked. It turns out, the longer the bread was cooked the longer it stayed in the stomach. Furthermore, the over-baked bread caused an immune response in the bloodstream and was treated as a foreign invader.

In contrast, according to a 2018 study published in the journal *Frontiers in Psychology*, eating raw vegetables may help boost mental health and relieve symptoms of depression. Researchers of this study found that people who consumed more produce in its natural, uncooked state reported higher levels of psychological well-being compared to those who ate mostly cooked alternatives.[77]

As perhaps one of the most interesting researchers and scientists to uncover the power of raw food, Francis Pottenger discovered that every food has a heat labile point (the temperature at which the chemical configuration of food changes). To determine this Pottenger conceived of an experiment in which one group of cats received only raw milk and raw meat, while other groups received part of the diet as pasteurized milk or cooked meat.

To Pottenger's amazement, he found that only those cats whose diet was totally raw survived an adrenalectomy. As his research progressed, he also noticed that only the all-raw group continued in good health generation after generation with excellent bone structure, freedom from parasites and vermin, easy pregnancies and gentle dispositions.

In contrast, all of the group whose diet was partially cooked, developed "facial deformities" of the exact same kind that Dr. Weston A. Price observed in human groups including narrowed faces, crowded jaws, frail bones and weakened ligaments.

The cats that ate cooked foods were also plagued with parasites, developed all manner of diseases and had difficult pregnancies. Female cats even became aggressive while the males became docile. After just three generations, young animals died before reaching adulthood and reproduction completely ceased.

Clearly, this is not very encouraging if you're eating a lot of cooked food and you may be wondering:

What's happening inside
during the digestion of cooked foods?

Studies show that the more food is cooked the longer it sits in your gut and the longer it sits in your gut the more it ferments. While eating fermented foods, which contain enzymes, breaks down hard to digest lectins and provides healthy bacteria, this type of fermentation is more like eating toxic food.

Remember, when you overcook food you kill off most exogenous enzymes. So while you still may have some endogenous enzymes, this compromises your ability to digest food, proteins start to putrefy and fats go rancid, irritating the mucosal lining of your gut and causing inflammation. The irritated cells of your digestive lining then spread allowing undigested and partially digested foods to pass through your gut wall.

Unfortunately, this cycle can then lead to leaky gut syndrome, which is linked to many allergic, autoimmune and digestive conditions as mentioned earlier from the lectin power drains.

The first doctor to test and document the effects of cooked versus raw food on the immune system was Dr. Paul Kouchakoff of Switzerland. In the 1930s Kouchakoff found that food that was cooked until well done initiated a white blood cell rise called "digestive leukocytosis." Digestive leukocytosis resembles a stress response to infection or trauma. This increase in white blood cells had been observed by others but was thought to be a normal reaction to eating.

Let's just pause for a second to grasp the reality of this discovery.   Basically, when you eat food that has been overcooked or you just eat a lot of cooked food it's kind of like stabbing yourself with a knife or taking a hammer to your fingers and crushing them one by one. Your body has to go into emergency mode to repair the damage.

Fortunately, here's the good news: After a further study at the Institute of Chemical Chemistry, Kouchakoff and others found that unaltered food (food that was raw or heated at very low temperatures) did not cause this immune reaction. They found that only food heated at very high temperatures or food that was processed and refined caused this rise in white blood cells.

Because of this study, the authors renamed the phenomenon "pathological leukocytosis" because they deemed it abnormal (or more appropriately, a response to abnormal food). The strongest food triggers of this reaction, heated or not, were processed and refined foods such as pasteurized and homogenized milk (thanks a lot, Louis), margarine, refined chocolate, sugar, candy, white flour, alcohol and table salt.

Oh yeah, and remember that not so yummy acrylamide stuff found in French fries? Leif Busk, of the Swedish National Food Administration, says that not only do overcooked starchy foods cause the formation of cancer-causing acrylamide but meats cooked at high temperatures do as well; as evidenced by the 20 cancer-causing heterocyclic amines (HCAs) found in such meats.

We mentioned the power draining side effects of barbequed, fried and well-done meats but its important to drive home how much over-cooking can drain your power and make you sick.

This was also discovered in another landmark study, which found a distinct connection between well-done meats, stomach cancer and increased risk of breast, colorectal and pancreatic cancer.[78]

Further research by Nancy Appleton, author of "Suicide by Sugar," reports that the average cancer risk due to amine exposure in cooked foods rises from 1 in 10,000 to 1 in 50 for people who regularly eat large amounts of well-done and flame-broiled conventional meats.

And while you may not (at least intentionally) want to top that steak off by smoking 600 cigarettes simultaneously, an additional study revealed just this effect after participants chawed down a 35 ounce charbroiled steak, which contains as much as 600 cigarettes worth of the cancer-causing compound benzopyrene (yuck!).[79]

Acidity Vs. Alkalinity

Another major power drain occurs from eating too many overly acidic foods.

If you're unfamiliar with the delicate balance between acidity vs. alkalinity, this refers to your pH balance, which means "potential of hydrogen" and varies throughout your body.

For example, the pH of your blood should remain between 7.35 and 7.45 in order to create homeostasis. This is the delicate balance of hydrogen essential for life, which also enables your body to detoxify a certain amount of cooked foods. This balance between acidity and alkalinity is so crucial if you deviate by just 1/10th of a percent you could go into a coma or die.

In regards to food, essentially, all foods can be measured as to their pH level with "0" being completely acidic (think battery acid or Coke) and "14" being completely alkaline (think broccoli sprouts and spinach).

Again, we need balance, so we'll be eating both acidic and alkaline foods but it's important to understand that studies show eating too many acidic foods leads to inflammation, impaired cognitive ability and various diseases like cancer, atherosclerosis and diabetes. [80]

Fortunately, there is much we can learn from some of the most highly respected advocates of an alkaline diet including Dr. Robert Young, author of "The pH Miracle" who declares:

"The New Biology Disease is not caused by external sources such as bacteria. Disease occurs within the body when acidity undermines the immune system. When our bodies are at the proper acid/alkaline balance, we can combat and defeat any invader, correct any imbalance, roll with all the punches. "

"Acidosis (too much acid in your blood), is due to environmental pollutants and stress, processed and refined foods, lack of biogenic or "life-giving" foods and mineral-deficient water, which contributes to disease and disorder within your body. The major cause of acidity is diet. Cooked foods create acidity in the body. Raw foods neutralize acid and are loaded with antioxidants."

Did you catch those last two sentences? Even if you didn't, I'll repeat them so you can remember this crucial lesson:

"Cooked foods create acidity in the body.
Raw foods neutralize acid and are loaded
with antioxidants."

At this point, I'd imagine you're probably wondering just how much acidic vs. alkaline food you need to eat in order to maximize your power and not get sick.

According to most experts, in order to clean out the acid and inflammation in your body and stay alkaline, the optimal ratio is around 3:1. In other words, you need to eat 3 alkaline foods (7 pH or above) for every 1 acidic food (Below 7 pH). So remember this one:

Eat 3 Alkaline Foods For Every 1 Acidic Food

To determine whether or not the foods you're eating are alkaline or I've listed the three main categories for acidic, neutral and alkaline. While this is not a complete list of foods, and you can download a free alkaline chart online,

this will give you an idea of how you are faring in your 3:1
balance of alkaline foods vs. acidic foods.

- **Acidic:** meat, poultry, fish, dairy, eggs, grains, alcohol

- **Neutral:** natural fats, starches, and sugars

- **Alkaline:** fruits, nuts, legumes (pressure cooked and
  sprouted), and vegetables

As you can see from the list above, some of your favorite
foods and beverages may not have possessed the alkaline
powers you predicted. But remember, we want balance;
specifically, a 3:1 balance of alkaline foods to acidic foods.

Beverages

Another striking discovery you may have noticed from this
chart is the power draining effect created by many common
beverages. And since water consumption is a significant
piece of the power puzzle, we'll need to dial this one in.

As you can see from the chart, the most acidic beverages
are carbonated water, club soda, energy drinks and soda
pop. And if you love America's most favorite beverages,
Coca Cola or Pepsi, I have some good and bad news.

First the bad news: both barely register on our chart,
weighing in at a dismal 2.3 pH level. And while you may not
think that's a big deal, when you consider the fact that each
whole pH value below 7 is ten times more acidic than the
next higher value, you'll start to grasp the massive potential
for disaster here.

For example, a pH of 3 is ten times more acidic than
a pH of 4 and 100 times more acidic than a pH of 5.

Sadly, that Coke you may or may not be drinking could
more aptly be related to battery acid than a power producing
beverage.

But this is just the beginning as these beverages also
include that omnipresent creator of inflammation called
"sugar!" Of course, excess sugar jacks up your insulin and
not only leads to inflammation but heart disease, diabetes,

and obesity. To top it off, combining sugar with carbonation creates severe tooth decay.[81]

What about fruit juice?

While you may think that natural fruits are safe to slog down in some form of condensed fruit juice, you should also understand that these contain highly concentrated amounts of fructose, a sugar that when consumed in excessive quantities can also lead to insulin resistance, diabetes and obesity.[82 83 84]

And if that isn't enough to convince you to give up or at least cut down those concentrated fruit juices you may want to consider the fact that any amount of fructose consumption increases appetite and promotes overeating.[85]

What about carbonated water?

You may have also noticed carbonated water didn't exactly score huge points in pH power but unless there is sugar in your carbonated beverage this is not something to be overly concerned about. According to studies, plain sparkling water does not appear to pose any health risks, only the ones with sugar do.[86] This is because your kidneys and lungs remove excess carbon dioxide, which then keeps your blood at a slightly alkaline level.

Additionally, if you drink beverages like Pellegrino, which comes from a natural spring source, you'll find they have much higher pH levels due to their natural mineral content (Pellegrino has a 5.6 pH level).

What about alkaline water?

Current trends promote buying commercial water with super high pH levels of 8.8 or higher. These products contain a high amount of dissolved minerals like calcium, potassium, and magnesium and can actually drain your power. This may sound contradictory but it relates back to the delicate balance of your microbiome.

According to New York Times bestselling author and world-renowned health expert, Dr. Sarah Ballantyne, Ph.D. (aka The Paleo Mom):

"Probiotic species are adapted to an acidic environment, and in fact produce organic acids, like lactic acid and butyric acid, that help control the growth of pathogens by lowering the pH of the intestines."

While you need calcium, salt, potassium, and magnesium to boost your alkalinity, unfortunately, these alkaline waters neutralize your stomach acid needed to digest your food. As Dr. Ballantyne continues:

"Studies also confirm that drinking alkaline water causes an undesirable shift in gut microbiome composition. A randomized, controlled crossover intervention in adult men compared the impact on the gut microbiome of consuming 2 liters per day of alkaline water (pH 9) compared to neutral water (pH 7) for two weeks. While the alkaline water had no effect on overall species diversity or richness, the men benefited from higher hydration levels from neutral pH water, which significantly increased richness by 15% when comparing pre- and post-intervention samples."

In contrast to these highly alkaline products, you may have noticed that the natural water sources on our chart run slightly acidic to just slightly alkaline.

So while you may want to stay away from these highly alkaline commercial waters, especially when you are digesting food, you can get a power boost from adding natural minerals to your water or buying water that has natural mineral content.

This is especially true if you've been eating acidic foods or have an abnormal amount of stress from work, relationships or illness and need to boost your alkalinity.

Minerals / Electrolytes / Hydration

Regardless of your circumstances, these minerals like potassium, sodium, calcium and magnesium raise your pH level, make you more alkaline and help you remain hydrated. As such, you should add minerals to your diet regularly.

This can be achieved quite simply by adding a pinch of Himalayan pink salt to your power meals as well as drinking water. Dr. Dominique D'Agostino, founder of Keto Nutrition, recommends 1-2 teaspoons per day as a healthy level of consumption.

And if you're not already hip to the Himalayan stuff, you'll be surprised to learn that it contains a full spectrum of 84 minerals including calcium, magnesium, potassium, copper and iron. So by adding the pink stuff to your food and water, you'll not only get an instant boost in alkalinity but the salt will also help you retain water and stay hydrated.

In contrast, if you chug a big glass of water with no minerals you'll most likely just pee most of it out within a short period of time.

Keep in mind; regular table salt does not do this. In fact, regular table salt is a power drain, which you should avoid. This is due to the fact that table salt is highly processed and the balance of sodium in comparison to other valuable minerals is lost.

In addition to mineral loss, anti-caking agents are added, which contain carcinogenic aluminum and can accumulate in your brain and lead to neurological diseases such as Alzheimer's.[87] [88]

Lastly, as an outdated practice, Iodine is also added to table salt to avoid goiters, which is no longer the crisis it was in the 1960s when companies began adding it.

Besides, if you are eating power boosting foods from *The Power Diet* you'll get plenty of iodine.

And if you're worried about all the hype around ingesting too much salt, you should know that the problems of hypertension and heart disease from overconsumption of salt is found primarily in people who have a diet high in processed table salt and processed foods, which contain way too much salt.[89] [90]

So if you're using processed table salt or eating a lot of packaged and processed products like potato chips, pizza, condiments, crackers, canned soups, lunchmeats, salted nuts and cheese you'll need to start eliminating these, as they will create inflammation and drain your power.

If you simply follow *The Power Diet* protocol you won't crave these power drains. Instead, you'll look forward to natural, nutrient dense, whole foods that are deeply satisfying and allow you to bypass the surgery (pun intended) that results from nutrient deficiencies or overconsumption of salt.

To maintain alkalinity, again you can simply add a pinch of Himalayan sea salt to your meals and when you drink water you can do the same thing and/or add lemon or lime or trace minerals.

How much should I drink per day?

As for water consumption recommendations, make sure you stick to natural mineral water or filtered water and avoid tap water as it is typically loaded with chlorine and fluoride, two massive power drains, which can lead to bladder and bone cancer.[91] [92]

Specifically, you should aim for .5 to 1 ounce per pound of body weight per day. So for example, if you weighed 150 pounds, normal consumption would be anywhere between 10 and 20 cups of water (8 ounces = 1 cup).

Now let's recap what we know about the power drains and power boosters.

> ✓ **Power Drain:** Overly acidic beverages with sugar like soda pop, coca cola, energy drinks like red bull, and concentrated fruit juices.

> ✓ **Power Boost:** Water from natural spring sources, filtered tap water, carbonated beverages sourced from natural springs, filtered water with lemon/lime or natural trace minerals added, green drinks with low to no sugar.

Megahertz Energy

When we talk about power, most people think about the power to influence people, run really fast, bench press 300 pounds or turn your lights on in your house. So when I tell people their food has power, they typically look perplexed and ask: "what do you mean?"

While this may be news to you, the amount of power contained in food, just like many other things in life, can be measured. Specifically, food can be measured in megahertz (MHz), a scientific measurement of the frequency and vibration of energy.

Similar to computers and electronic devices, our bodies require specific ranges of megahertz of energy to function properly and operate at their best.

For example, cellular activity in your body requires an optimal range of approximately 60 – 70 megahertz of energy to function properly. It may be of no surprise then that research has shown cysts, diseases, infections and tumors typically occur when tissues are below 50 MHz of energy.[93]

What's important to understand here is that megahertz levels can be found throughout your body, cells, glands, organs and nervous system and they begin to malfunction when you feed them with foods that provide less than 60 – 70 MHz. And once your body and its organs go below 60 MHz, your digestive, immune and nervous systems begins to slow down and reduce their proper functions, which in turn, drains power and leads to illness and disease.

Biophotons

Adding more sunshine to the darkness of dead food is the fact that plant materials soak up and store photons (particles of light which carry energy) radiated by the sun, transforming them into "Biophotons," a term coined in the 1970s by German scientist Fritz-Albert Popp.

Popp followed up on the work of Russian scientist, Alexander Gurwitsch, who discovered that all living things emit photons within the ultraviolet range of the spectrum and concluded that DNA is a major source of these emissions.

By developing a device that could measure these very low-level light waves he discovered that the emissions from healthy people are significantly stronger than those from people who are ill.

But even more impressive is what he found when he evaluated the biophotons in food. What he found was that organic foods gave off five times as much biophotonic energy as commercially grown foods and cooked or irradiated food emitted virtually no biophotons. And since biophotons possess the power to energize and heal those who consume them *The Power Diet* enthusiastically includes a healthy dose of raw organic foods.

What Foods Drain or Boost Power?

Predictably, with rare exceptions, the same Power Draining Foods mentioned earlier are also low on megahertz and the same Power Boosting Foods are high in megahertz. This is good news since you won't have to memorize another list.

That being said, it's important to understand where some of these foods fall on the megahertz measurement scale. So let's take a look at some examples.

Just make sure you ask yourself what happened the last time you ate each one of these foods, not just from the immediate sugar rush but an hour or two down the road. Did you feel more or less energy?

✓ Refined Processed French fries, waffles, donuts, potato chips, candy, alcohol, white bread = 0 - 5 MHz

✓ Cooked Meat = 2 - 10 MHz

✓ Fresh herbs = 20 - 27 MHz

✓ Green foods = 65 - 75 MHz

✓ Green fresh/cold-pressed juice and spirulina = 170 MHz

More often than not, what you'll experience after eating high megahertz foods combined with *The Power Diet* fats and proteins is a sustained boost of energy for two hours or more. In contrast, low megahertz low alkalinity foods will give a quick sugar rush then drop you off a cliff and send you to the couch within an hour or two.

So if you're feeling tired but you're well rested and you're not fighting an illness, there's a really good chance you're eating power draining low megahertz foods.

And while raw green foods provide the most megahertz power, shifting towards a 100% plant based diet may not work for everyone long-term. For this reason, I recommend focusing more on the ideal ratio of high and low megahertz foods that create an alkaline pH level and boost your overall power.

Fortunately, this ratio is identical to our alkaline vs. acid balance. So again, all you need to remember is the following:

Eat 3 Alkaline Foods For Every 1 Acidic Food

Note: It's important to understand that the more you cook meat and vegetables the lower the megahertz and the higher the acidity. In order to avoid the toxins and power drain of overcooking try steaming, low heat cooking or eating raw.

Recap of The Power Drains

It's time to celebrate because you've reached the end of the quality components of food and it's now time to move on to our second pillar - quantity. But before we do let's recap what you've learned so far about the Power Drains so you remember what to eliminate and avoid in the future.

As mentioned earlier, this is highly significant, since your primary focus should be to remove the power draining foods and restore the delicate balance of your microbiome. If you can do this, your body will naturally restore itself back to full power and you can eat without worrying much about your weight or your energy levels.

Stay Away From Food That Contains Any Of These Power Drains:

- ✓ Toxic herbicides and pesticides

- ✓ Unnatural Preservatives & Additives

- ✓ GMO's

- ✓ Artificial sweeteners

- ✓ Hydrogenated oils (trans fats)

- ✓ Over processed and refined foods

- ✓ Toxic lectins found primarily in grains and legumes (some exceptions can be pressure cooked, sprouted or fermented)

- ✓ Highly acidic foods

- ✓ Overcooked foods (fried, grilled, broiled, etc.)

Take Action – Eliminate Low Quality Food

Again, repetition is the mother of all skill, so let's go ahead and repeat the action steps for eliminating power draining food but this time we'll add in our two additional power drains. Take note and remember that there are 4 critical power drains that you need to pay special attention to and begin eliminating from your diet.

Limit or Eliminate The 4 Power Drains

1) **Limit or Eliminate Processed Foods** - Packaged, canned and processed foods drain your power. Eat organic whole foods whenever possible.

2) **Read Labels** - If you do buy something that was modified or processed from its original state read the label. If you can't understand an ingredient it's most likely toxic and

you should avoid it. If it doesn't have a label ask the vendor, **"What's in it?"**

3) **Limit or Remove Toxic Antinutrients** - Start limiting toxic antinutrients like oxalates and tannins and removing power draining lectins out of your diet for 30 days and notice if you feel a power boost.

4) **Eat More Raw Food & Stop Overcooking** - Boost your alkalinity and megahertz energy by cutting back on cooked food and eating more raw foods. Stick to the 3:1 ratio of 3 alkaline (high megahertz) foods to 1 acidic (low megahertz) food.

Buy A Steamer

To stop overcooking make sure you buy a steamer if you don't already own one. This will help you immensely in avoiding overcooking food as well as breaking down hard to digest foods like cruciferous vegetables (see Resources for recommendations).

Beverage Boost Twice A Day

Make sure you boost your alkalinity immediately when you wake up in the morning by drinking a glass of clean water with ½ to 1 whole fresh squeezed lemon or lime. Then when you start to hit the skids and feel tired in the afternoon do the same thing or add a scoop of antioxidant powder (see "Power Supplements" for recommendations). This will boost your energy so you don't need coffee or a nap, (unless you're sleeping less than 7 hours a day, in which case you may need a short nap).

Test Your Alkalinity

To test your alkalinity, buy some alkalinity strips. These only cost a few dollars and can reveal some startling truths about the darkness of too much dead food in your diet. For affordable recommendations on all these items check our resources page at:
www.ChadScottCoaching.com/resources

Pillar 2 – Quantity

Once you're eating clean and toxin free foods, the next most obvious trap people fall prey to is simply eating too much.

Arguably the most obvious occasion that highlights this challenge occurs during the Holidays. Typically, there are plenty of parties to go to, lots of treats to eat, and no shortage of comfort food, which makes overeating difficult to avoid.

For most of my life, I followed this pattern. I would fill up my plate until there wasn't any room on it. I would cover everything with acrylamide laden gravy, slap on a heap of Grandma's famous green beans loaded with gut bulging lectins on top of an overcooked acidic turkey and stuffing made of corn and wheat loaded with acid forming antinutrients.

And let's not forget about dessert. I had to try every dessert, including the apple pie topped with pasteurized A1 casein ice cream and some chocolate pecan pie loaded with so much sugar it made my insulin spike through the roof and my gut bulge like I was pregnant.

I would eat until I simply couldn't eat anymore, which taxed my digestive system to the point of bloating, gas, reflux (heartburn) and stomach pain.

Of course, I made attempts to temper the inner explosions of inflammation with antacids and enzyme supplements but it made very little difference. I would then go to bed, have crazy disturbing dreams, wake up and do it all over again until the damn holidays were finally over.

Low and behold, around one week later I would find myself hacking my brains out with the flu or a nasty cold that made me miserable and useless for another week or two. Despite the pain and discomfort I, like so many others, continued to overeat every year regardless of the price.

While this may or may not be a typical Holiday scenario for you, it proves a point - overeating drains your power and puts you back on the couch.

Fortunately, by mindfully manipulating macronutrient ratios we can remove the power drains, stop overeating and feel like a million bucks, even in the aftermath of the holidays. And if it's any consolation, I've been faithfully following *The Power Diet* for the last seven years now and haven't had to suffer from the flu since.

Macronutrients

Pillar #2 is all about Macronutrients (AKA Macros). This includes fat, protein, and carbohydrates, which are the primary elements that make up a food's composition and help you create energy and power. You can find them listed on the nutrition facts panel of most foods or by using online apps and calculators.

Macros are then comprised of calories or "units of energy." What's important to understand about macros is that not all calories are equal.

For instance, one gram of carbohydrates or protein provides 4 calories, while one gram of fat provides 9 calories. As you can see, fat provides more than twice as many calories as either carbs or protein. This is good news because you'll be eating mostly fat on *The Power Diet*.

Why Counting Calories Doesn't Work

One of the oldest and most outdated nutritional practices is "calories in calories out" (CICO), which has been pounded into the nutritional mainstream for centuries. The idea is that by simply eating fewer calories than you burn you will lose weight and visa versa.

The problem with CICO alone is that it won't tell you the balance of fat, carbohydrates, and protein in the foods you eat, which is a crucial mistake that could have seriously damaging repercussions.

For example, let's say you want to lose weight and you go on a vegetarian diet and unknowingly eat 60% of your calories from carbohydrates (which is quite common). This will have a massively different effect on your weight, power and energy than if you had eaten 60% of your diet from healthy fat sources.

As best selling author Dr. Joe Mercola says, "fat for fuel" is a far superior source of sustained energy than carbohydrates.

Additionally, according to experts like Dave Asprey, CICO does not take into consideration the effect of macros on your hormones, which have been shown to affect weight gain completely independent of the amount of calories consumed.

Thankfully, in *The Power Diet,* you won't have to bang your head against the wall or break out your calculator and count calories every time you need to eat a meal. Instead, we'll go beyond counting calories and focus on tracking macros, a much more effective and reliable strategy that takes into consideration the individual effects of carbs, protein, fat and their effect on your hormones.

Mindful Eating

In my experience, most people (I've been guilty), approach a meal thinking something along the lines of: "I need some kind of protein and starch and what salad or veggie would go good with that."

What they do not realize is that some of these foods may be draining power by over or under consuming a particular macro.

For example, I used to mindlessly put together a veggie bowl with some fish with no thought as to how much carbs, fat and protein were really optimal. Of course, I never really felt that amazing after eating it either. Instead, I felt drained of power and needed to take a nap an hour or two later.

But once I really got committed to maximizing power and feeling really good, I slowed down and became more mindful by measuring the grams of carbs, fats and protein in each one of the ingredients in my food. What I realized was that I was way off, and in some instances, I was eating twice as much protein and carbs as I needed.

This was a huge revelation for me and doubled my power once I cut back on the protein and carbs. So I want to encourage you right now to stop mindlessly throwing food on a plate or ordering something just because it looks good and slow down to mindfully think about what you are eating; then ask yourself our master question:

Does This Food Give Me Power Or Take It Away?

While you won't be counting calories on *The Power Diet*, initially, it's super important you understand and get familiar with how many grams of a particular macro is included in each food you are eating.

To assist you in this process I'll offer examples later on and I encourage you to check out our <u>video library</u> where you can find step-by-step instructions on how to build power meals quickly (under 10 minutes) so eventually, you will not have to measure the grams in your macros. All you'll need to do is simply eyeball the food and you'll be good to go.

Realistically, this will take a good 2-4 weeks of consistent practice. So be patient and just know, this is a game changer strategy, which will completely change your life, with more energy, power and joy for the rest of your life.

Lastly, depending on your health goals, you can adjust the ratios of macronutrients you consume to lose weight, build muscle, or enter maintenance & expansion mode. More on mindful eating in a bit, for now, let's take a look at some of the other awesome power boosting effects of balancing macros to make sure you invest in this strategy long-term.

Big Benefits of Balancing Macros

Flexibility

Ultra-stringent diets that require you to laboriously count calories can lead to frustration, cravings, and eventual failure. Let's face it, when you're hungry, at a restaurant or having fun at a party, who wants to count calories?

In contrast, the flexibility of balancing macros in *The Power Diet* allows you to fall out of your target range for a bit without falling apart then bounce back quite quickly. There is no one size fits all here, instead, our goal is to get close to a target ratio and monitor whether or not your power is drained or boosted, then adjust accordingly.

It's More Enjoyable

Balancing your macros does not force you to eliminate entire food groups like carbohydrates. Instead, when you feel depleted or drained, again, you simply shift more or less from one of the three macros into the others.

It Prevents You From Overeating

Balancing your macros also helps to avoid some of the problems with overeating in one macro category. For example, I used to have a gardener who would eat refried beans and corn tortillas for lunch every day and literally within 15 minutes he would fall asleep in his chair. Why?

No, it's not because all Latin Americans need a siesta, it's because beans and corn tortillas have some of the highest carbohydrate and lectin content of any foods and anyone who eats them is going to be severely drained of power.

Or let's say you eat way too much fat from coconut oil, avocados and sardines but very little carbs or vegetables. In this case, you may feel constipated simply because you aren't getting enough fiber. Unfortunately, counting calories will never explain why you're so backed up.

Helps Manage and Reverse Chronic Diseases

Managing and avoiding disease by balancing your macros isn't just hearsay. Researchers have proven scientifically that managing macros can help boost your health on multiple fronts as well as reverse conditions such as diabetes,[94] certain cancers,[95] and polycystic ovary syndrome.[96]

The Power Drain Dilemma

Yes, balancing your macros can be a game changer but only if you can leap over the mountain of carbohydrates that flood our markets, kitchens, restaurants and vending machines.

Look around the next time you go to the store or a friend's house and what you'll most likely see is the predominance of some kind of food (or fake food) made primarily of carbohydrates.

Of course, there's a reason (even if isn't good) for this proliferation of carbs: they instantly make you feel good!

It's no big secret that carbohydrates stimulate the production of feel good chemicals like serotonin. And since we are pleasure seeking, pain avoiding creatures, carbs supply a quick hit of instant gratification.

To make matters worse, nutritionists, doctors and the government have been telling us to eat a diet high in complex carbohydrates and low in saturated fats for decades.

Irresponsibly, these so-called experts have been recommending upwards of 50% to 60% of daily calories be consumed from carbohydrates - even to those with diabetes and inflammatory diseases.

Adding fuel to the mounting inflammation, we are bombarded (quite publicly) by these so-called experts' incessant campaigns to demonize healthy high-fat foods and its advocates who have helped millions of people regain their health.

Regrettably, this advice is the exact opposite of what a person with diabetes (or anyone) needs to reach optimal health and… the facts speak for themselves.

There is no shortage of studies proving that the shift to a more grain-based diet has led to increased rates of obesity, diabetes, and chronic diseases, including a 14-year study involving 27,000 people between ages 45 and 74.

In this study, researchers found that those who consumed eight servings of full-fat dairy products a day cut their risk of diabetes by 25% compared to those who ate fewer servings.[97]

An additional study published in 2010 also suggested that palmitoleic acid, which naturally occurs in full-fat dairy products, protects against insulin resistance and diabetes.[98]

Athletic Performance

As a lifetime athlete, I've always been curious about what the top athletes in the world are using to boost their performance. And while you may not be an elite athlete, there is much we can learn from a community that spends a big chunk of their time optimizing diet to maximize power and performance.

In a study published in the journal, Medicine & Science in Sports & Exercise, researchers reported that 31% of elite Ironman triathlon competitors experienced serious gastrointestinal distress during their event.

According to veteran endurance athlete and best selling author Mark Sisson:

"All long and ultra endurance athletes experience at least mild digestive issues in attempting the impossible task of processing sugary calories while blood has been shunted away from digestive organs."

Further, Mark points to some striking examples of elite athletes like Sami Inkinen, a world champion amateur triathlete who was able to extend his burnout time (glucose depletion) from 5.6 hours to 87 hours after transitioning from a traditional higher carb eating pattern to a fat and keto adapted eating pattern.

An additional study conducted by Dr. Volek, et. all dubbed "FASTER" (Fat Adapted Substrate oxidation in Trained Elite Runners) revealed that low-carb endurance athletes easily access and burn significantly more fat than high-carbohydrate endurance athletes.

This is significant since it places less reliance on external fuel sources of carbs, which minimizes digestive issues, and depletion of glucose. By burning mostly fat, the low carb athletes also didn't suffer the severe glycogen depletion of high carb athletes who needed massive high carb recovery feeding. As Sisson says:

"When you gorge on a big meal after a workout, you increase oxidative stress to the gastrointestinal system,

*potentially delaying recovery and increasing the overall
stress impact of the workout and the eating binge… if you
overwhelm it (your liver) with frequent carb slams, you can
compromise your ability to recover from exercise and all
other forms of stress."*

But what about carbs for recovery?

If you still believe you need massive carbohydrate intake in
order to manage recovery from exercise consider elite ultra-
runner Zach Bitter. As the USA national 100k champion who
was part of the FASTER Study, Zack was able to complete
an 8.5 hour 38 mile endurance run through river canyons in
the Sierra Nevada mountains while consuming only water
and liquid amino acids.

It turns out, these same studies show that a low-carb
high-fat diet like *The Power Diet* enables you to recover from
exercise much more efficiently than a high-carb low fat-diet
whether it's a 100 mile run, a power lift, a sprint down the
field or any other exercise.

Lastly, this same study showed that while both high carb
and low carb athletes had significantly depleted their
glycogen stores after three hours on the treadmill, the low
carb athletes were able to restock glycogen even more
efficiently than the high carb athletes, despite consuming
extremely minimal post-exercise carbohydrates.

The Real Culprit Of Power Drain

Clearly healthy fat is not the main thing draining your power.
The real culprit of low performance, inflammation, diabetes,
weight gain and most of today's diseases is the
overconsumption of carbohydrates, especially the refined
varieties. This overconsumption, in turn, creates insulin
resistance and sets off a chain reaction of sabotaging
effects.

Regrettably, when you eat too many carbs, over time,
cells in your muscles, body fat, and liver start resisting or
ignoring the signal that the hormone **insulin** is trying to send

out, which is to grab glucose from your bloodstream and put it into your cells to use as energy.

Once your cells become desensitized to the frequent surges of insulin and cannot use it as fuel, this glucose gets stored as fat and can eventually lead to inflammatory diseases and obesity.

The 2.5 Million Year Old Fad Diet - Metabolic Flexibility

Fortunately, in *The Power Diet,* we'll be using what is called "Metabolic Flexibility," which means your body will use primarily fat for fuel with the added flexibility of burning carbs and protein as glucose (sugar), or glycogen (sugar stores).

Again, there's a really good reason for this strategy and it dates back to a time prior to the availability of Carbo laden treats from McDonalds, Dunkin Donuts or Coca Cola; a time when most people were metabolically flexible by necessity.

For example, 300 thousand years ago a tribe of cave dwellers set out on the migration trail and killed a deer, which gave them sustenance for weeks. And while the following month they may have experienced famine (with no 7-11 or Coca Cola), fortunately, metabolic flexibility allowed them to burn stored fat as ketones and feel fine even if they didn't eat.

Ketones are chemicals made by your liver when you don't have enough insulin to turn sugar (aka glucose) into energy. But this is a good thing since too much insulin from eating too many carbs leads to insulin resistance and diabetes both of which are high risk factors for death from COVID-19.

Fortunately, when insulin is low, because you are "metabolically flexible," your liver turns fat into ketones, which supplies your body and mind with high powered, long lasting fuel. Essentially, as diet that focuses on burning ketones The Power Diet is considered a "ketogenic diet."

The problem, as explained by Dr. Joseph Mercola is this:

"With today's standard American diet, most people never reach this state of fat burning and ketosis. They're constantly feeding their bodies carbohydrates, and in this high-insulin state, they simply cannot burn fat. Over time, it wears out

your metabolic machinery, resulting in insulin resistance and weight gain." [99]

Essentially, what this means that by implementing The Power Diet you can limit if not eliminate two of the biggest risk factors for hospitalization and death from COVID-19 and other illness that are caused by insulin resistance and diabetes.

And if, for any reason, you've heard this ketogenic type of diet labeled as a "fad diet" think again. Our species has been eating keto for over 2.5 million years. In contrast, humans have been eating grains for roughly 10,000 years.

This should be really good news, especially if you are overly dependent on carbs and feel like a slave to food; like you need to eat every couple hours to keep from getting hungry, grumpy, and losing focus.

Are You A Carboholic?

This brings us to our next big question:

Can you get addicted to carbs (AKA carboholic)?

I met a woman from Persia who told me how she couldn't live without rice and how she loved the taste so much better than cauliflower rice. She believed it was purely based on taste preference.

But what she did not know was that each time she became hungry a hormone called "ghrelin" was activated to signal to her stomach and brain that it was time to eat. Since ghrelin crosses the blood brain burier and stimulates hunger sensations in the hypothalamus (your brain's control center for impulse control, decision making and emotions like anger and pleasure) her hungry hypothalamus was most likely ditching her more disciplined behavior and opting to answer the intense hunger call with an infusion of carbohydrates from rice.

To put this into perspective, according to best selling author of "The Primal Blueprint" Mark Sisson, this gal's actions would in turn:

"Trigger a burst of dopamine and endogenous opioids that act on the nucleus accumbens in the hypothalamus to influence neural mediation of food reward; you form a strong connection in the pleasure center of your brain between carbohydrates and intense reward. The fact that sugar and wheat has additional opioid stimulating properties strengthens this connection. What's more Dr. Cate asserts that cortisol is a further trigger for habit-forming associations. When you're stressed – whether by exercise induced depletion or by hassles of daily life - and you consume sugar, your brain is cementing a connection between stress and sugar. The incessant burning of and refueling of carbs locks you into a hormonal and psychological carbohydrate dependency pattern..."

Question: Do you know of someone, perhaps intimately, who may be dependent on carbs?
Personally I'm well fat adapted and don't struggle with this anymore but I realized how much of a challenge it is for many when recently visiting my brother and his family.

My brother is my identical twin and while we share the same diet, the rest of his family does not. So when he threw away his daughter's three-day-old wheat pizza a tenuous battle erupted in what is, with rare exception, a very calm, tranquil, and loving environment.

At first, I was amused to watch someone so upset over something so trivial as pizza until I remembered the drug like effects of wheat, which triggers the same opioid receptors as heroin. [100] [101]

This is a serious challenge, so if you experience frequent cravings for carbohydrates like potato chips, pizza, crackers, soda and high carb snacks, just know you could be hard wired to crave carbs.

Similar to a drug addict, when you don't get your carbs, your body joneses for them, and you're stuck with cravings, low blood sugar and lack of focus until you get your fix.

Even worse, these excess carbs create inflammation and an environment that encourages the proliferation of harmful pathogens, bacteria and viruses. This obviously drains your power and more than likely sets you up for illness and disease (remember the holidays?). And since I'm pretty sure you're reading this because you want to increase your power and feel amazing the real question here is this:

How can I break the chains of slavery to carbohydrates and boost my power?

Ketosis Can Unleash Maximum Power

If you really want to unleash maximum power both mentally and physically, the answer to this question and your new goal for the rest of your life should be this:

**I am committed to burning fat
as my primary fuel source!**

To achieve this we'll be optimizing two of our three key variables "Quantity" & "Frequency."

First, by increasing fat intake and lowering both carbs and protein we'll optimize the first variable "Quantity" so you turn into a lean, mean, fat burning machine! Of course, you could swap out "mean" with "clean" or "kind" but you get the point.

Second, to optimize your second variable "Frequency" and boost your fat burning ability even further, we'll be increasing the time you do not eat during the day.

By optimizing these two variables, your body will begin to shift towards "ketosis," a naturally occurring metabolic state where your body burns primarily fat for fuel. This will then begin to significantly lower your levels of insulin while fatty acids are released from your body fat stores to use as energy. And yes, if you're overweight that means shedding unwanted, unsightly fat (like butter on a hot frying pan).

And if for any reason you're at all apprehensive about giving up some of those carbs and eating less, don't worry;

The Power Diet offers plenty of calories and allows for flexibility in macro consumption.

And besides, the common myth that your brain needs 130 grams of carbs per day to function properly was debunked long ago. In fact, a report by the US Institute of Medicine's Food and Nutrition Board states:

"The lower limit of dietary carbohydrates compatible with life apparently is zero, provided that adequate amounts of protein and fat are consumed."[102]

Yes, a zero-carb diet could be achieved but it's considered extreme by most experts and it doesn't allow for the consumption of many healthy foods that feed your brain with glucose, which brings us to the next piece of the flexibility formula.

Since your brain cannot use fat as a fuel source, when your carb intake falls below roughly 50 grams per day, your liver produces ketones from fatty acids when glucose and insulin levels are low.[103]

But here's the catch, when carbs are eliminated or minimized, ketones can only provide roughly 70% of the brain's energy needs.[104]

Remember, we are trying to create long-term sustainability, which means being more flexible when it comes to recommending foods. Accordingly, *The Power Diet* offers a smart range of macro consumption depending on your circumstances and allows you to cycle in and out of ketosis by increasing your carbs and opening your eating window a couple of days a week.

This strategy has been used for hundreds of thousands of years by our ancestors and can go a long way in making *The Power Diet* more sustainable and enjoyable for you long-term.

Think of it this way: our metabolically flexible ancestors, more often than not, experienced feast or famine. So when a big score was made (killed a deer or found a beehive) they indulged, cycled out of ketosis and stored up calories for the impending lean times ahead.

Similarly, in modern times several factors could also warrant cycling out of ketosis, such as a birthday that features the most luscious banana cream pie with caramel infused chocolate or a night out on the town at a great Italian restaurant that features six cheese lasagna and garlic bread balls.

As long as you stick to The Power Diet protocol, you won't have to worry about indulging or celebrating from time to time. Just keep in mind, after you've been eating high-quality foods for a few months, when you do return to low quality, high sugar foods, you're body will feel the effects as a power drain.

To account for this and remain a happy eater, I'll give you some cleansing options, as well as some healthy treat recommendations that satisfy both your taste buds and boost your power.

While you can cycle off any day of the week, I recommend Saturday and Sunday, since these tend to be splurge days for most people. But again, *The Power Diet* is not a highly restrictive deprivation diet, which makes this completely optional. If you feel great and want to stick to your normal macro intake and frequency of eating, by all means, do.

In addition, there are some exceptions to the additional carb intake that could make this counterproductive. Notice if any of the following relate to you:

- I'm trying to lose weight
- I suffer from gut issues like leaky gut
- I'm just starting out and am having trouble becoming fat adapted and metabolically flexible

If you fit into these categories I recommend not adding in extra calories and sticking to the lower range of carbohydrate recommendations (10-15% of total daily calories) until you can reach your ideal weight and rectify any health issues.

Power Boosting Benefits of Ketosis

If for any reason you still feel apprehensive about reducing your carb and protein intake, again, don't sweat it, because

I'm going to arm you with some more firepower to stay on track.

As you read the power boosting elements of ketosis below, instead of just reading them, imagine yourself enjoying the benefits and what that would mean for your life.

In other words, how would this make you feel if you obtained these benefits, what would you do differently and how would that change your future for the better.

In the personal development field, we call this "future pacing," which effectively creates the future in advance and in the process helps you commit to taking the action necessary to make it happen. This is a powerful tool I use in all my mindset trainings including "<u>The Winner's Mindset</u>," which helps expedite changes like boosting your power and completely transforming your ability to step up and succeed in all areas of life.

If you struggle with self-discipline and taking the action necessary to create major life transformation, I highly recommend you check out that program at: www.ChadScottCoaching.com

Now let's envision some crucial wins in your life.

The Log vs. The stick

One of the best analogies for highlighting the difference and advantage of burning fat vs. carbs as your primary fuel source is the log vs. the stick.

When you're burning primarily carbs and you're glucose dependent, its sort of like throwing match sticks on a campfire. As time passes you have to constantly throw another stick in the fire to keep it going.

A typical match stick looks like a bread stick, potato chip, sports drink, soda pop, fruit, pastry, granola bar or candy bar (how long does Snickers really satisfy?).

In contrast, when you have become fat adapted and burn fat as your primary fuel source it's like throwing a big log on the fire. As time passes, it just keeps on burning - sure and steady. This log shows up as an avocado, walnuts, almonds, olive oil, coconut oil, fish, the perfect keto bar, etc.

Now can you imagine yourself as a stick that burns up in minutes or would you rather be a slow burning log that takes hours to burn?

More Testosterone

Remember those hormones we talked about, which CICO doesn't take into consideration? Well, testosterone is one of them, so if you're at all short on sexual potency I'd imagine this might be of special interest to you. Fortunately, the lists of studies on this subject are extensive as best selling author and well-known keto advocate Dave Asprey explains:

"Restricting calories and/or fat consumption, sends the same stress signals that shut down fertility and tells your body to use all your hormone building blocks to produce cortisol instead of testosterone… high cortisol produces insulin resistance, fat gain, and breakdown of muscle."

In one particular study participants who ingested 75 grams of glucose saw a decrease in testosterone levels by up to 25% for over two hours.[105] Of course, this makes sense when you consider corn flakes and graham crackers were designed to lower libido in a time when sex drive was considered a problem.

Fortunately, studies show that increasing saturated fat can actually increase your testosterone levels, the inverse of which has also been proven.

For example, when subjects who had been eating a diet consisting of over 40% fat reduced their consumption to 25% they found a corresponding decline in testosterone levels.[106] Imagine that, you get to eat fat and become sexually potent at the same time! Can you picture it?

While this may sound pretty awesome, just know, as all things in life have a limit, so too does fat consumption and its ability to boost your testosterone. Studies also show that by eating too much fat you can lower your testosterone, so make sure you follow *The Power Diet* guidelines for macronutrients.

No More Carboholic Cravings

By eating more fat and fewer carbs, over time, your body will adjust and gain more metabolic flexibility. And more importantly, you'll no longer be a slave to carbs and all their power draining effects like inflammation, cravings, low energy, poor focus and reduced power.

Can you imagine not having to constantly eat food or lose focus when you're doing something important?

Oxidative Damage Is Significantly Reduced

Free radicals are unstable atoms that can cause damage to parts of cells such as proteins, DNA, and cell membranes through a process called oxidation.

Unfortunately, when you burn primarily carbs as fuel (you're a stick burner), this raises your blood glucose levels too high and makes you more susceptible to the ravaging effects of oxidation.

In this regard, you can also think of carbs as dirty fuel that is more susceptible to oxidation and fat as clean burning fuel, which is less susceptible. As Dr. Joseph Mercola states:

"When you adopt a high-fat, low-carb diet and make the switch to burning fat and ketones for fuel instead of glucose, your mitochondria's exposure to oxidative damage drops by as much as 30 to 40 percent compared to when your primary source of fuel is sugar, as is typical in American diets today. This means that when you are "fat adapted"—that is, when you have made the transition to burning fat for fuel—your mitochondrial DNA, cell membranes, and protein can remain stronger, healthier, and more resilient."

This discovery is monumental since your mitochondria are the critical energy generating machines in every cell of your body. And the more mitochondria you have and the better they function the more powerful you'll be and the longer you'll live.

Now can you imagine having millions upon millions of little soldiers with protective shields over them cranking out power for you? This is the power provided by burning primarily fat instead of carbs.

Lose Weight & Stop Overeating

We mentioned this earlier but it's important you understand that studies consistently show by cutting carbs and eating more protein and fat, people end up eating far fewer calories because it leads to an automatic reduction in appetite.[107]

Do you remember the last time you had guacamole and chips? How did it taste? And do you remember starting to feel full even before the main course came?

This satiation didn't come from the corn chips (remember lectins), it came from the avocado, which probably saved you from overeating and gaining weight.

Enjoyable Long-Term As A Lifestyle

One of the main reasons people feel miserable and eventually give up on diets is the restricting nature of the diet. In contrast, *The Power Diet* gives you the flexibility to eat generous amounts of good healthy fats that most people love while adding in moderate proportions of carbs and protein, which keeps you satiated and satisfied on all levels.

Can you imagine eating rich delicious foods for the rest of your life while maintaining your ideal weight with maximum power to achieve and accomplish anything you set your mind to? I'm going to assume that's a "yes," which means its time dive a little deeper into quantity.

Suggested Macronutrient Ratios

Now that you've imagined and seen your future burning high-octane keto logs on *The Power Diet*, it's time to break down just how much fat, carbs and protein you need to become metabolically flexible and create maximum power.

Remember, this is not a one size fits all program and depending on many factors including genetics, stress, body type, and goals, you may need more or less of certain macros than others.

The beauty of *The Power Diet* is that it gives you the flexibility to stay within a healthy range, so you don't have to worry about getting the percentage of fat, protein or carbs exactly right at every meal. That being said, if you are over or underweight, by using a modified program as outlined in the groundbreaking *Fired Up* fitness program, you can achieve your ideal weight much faster.

As the companion program to *The Power Diet, Fired Up* offers three fitness programs including weight loss, weight gain, and maintenance & expansion. If you're interested in expediting your journey to optimum power and ideal weight check out the following link:

www.ChadScottCoaching.com/fired-up

Cycling In And Out Of Ketosis

In *The Power Diet*, you'll want to spend at least 5 days in a cycle of high fat, with reduced carbs and protein. This will keep your body in fat burning mode for most of the week and allow you to use ketones as high-powered fuel.

For the remaining two days of the week, you have the flexibility to continue with the high fat diet or cycle off as previously mentioned.

Since females (especially those of reproductive age) are more sensitive to caloric restriction, this cycle off period is recommended for all women. We'll talk more about this in the 3rd Pillar "Frequency," for now just know… ladies, you need to push up to the higher recommended dosage of carbohydrate macros.

To best understand this distribution of macros check out the following pie charts for Maintenance and Expansion macros:

The Power Diet Macros

Choose any 5-7 days per week to eat primarily healthy fats and reduce carbs and protein.

✓ High Fat - 50-70% of calories from healthy fats
✓ Low Carbs - 10-30% of calories from carbs.
✓ Low Protein - 10-20% of calories from protein

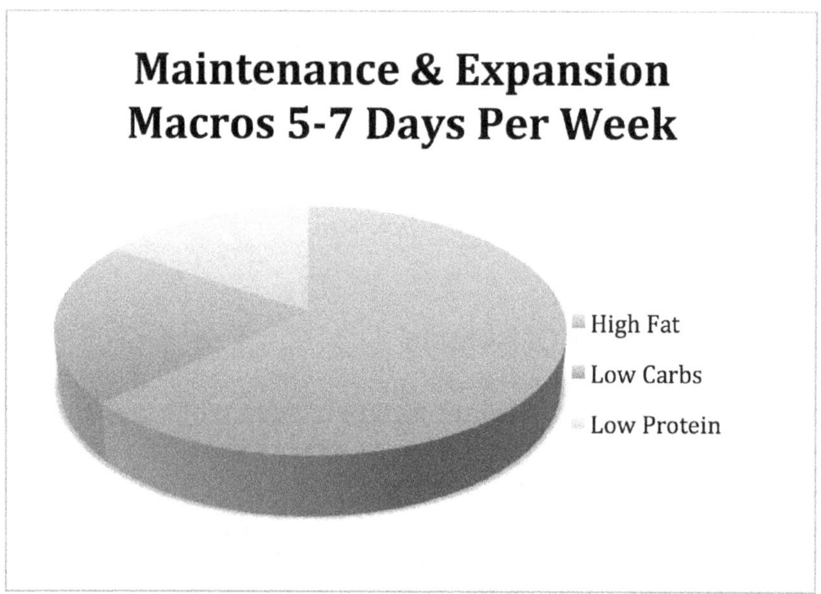

WARNING: Overconsumption Of Carbs Kills Power!

At this point, I need to issue a **warning**. As you may have noticed there is a wide range of fat and a smaller range for carbs and protein allotted in *The Power Diet*. This is due to the fact that once you have become metabolically flexible and adapted to burning fat as your primary fuel source you can eat more carbs and less fat without cycling out of ketosis.

So while most experts recommend eating less than 50 grams of carbs per day to burn a healthy amount of ketones and stay within a healthy blood glucose range, as a fat adapted person, I can eat over 100 grams of carbs no problem and according to my ketone blood test, still be burning a healthy amount of ketones with healthy blood glucose readings.

While part of this result is related to our third pillar "Frequency" the other part has to do with the fact that I'm well adapted to burning fat as my primary fuel source.

As such, when you're first starting out you will most likely not be able to burn fat as your primary fuel source (AKA "fat adapted"). **So listen closely:**

If you are not yet fat adapted and metabolically flexible (still dependent on throwing sticks on your campfire), you'll want to remain closer to the lower range of the carbohydrate ratio (10%-15%) and closer to the upper range or the fat ratio (60% - 70%).

The only exception to this is women. Since you ladies are by nature more sensitive to calorie restriction you can eat in the higher ranges of 15% to 30% carbs.

By sticking to high fat and low carb macros you will effectively accelerate your transition into burning fat (big logs) as your primary fuel source.

It's also important to understand that the biggest impact you can make in reducing your exposure to oxidative damage comes from keeping your blood glucose levels low, as evidenced by Dr. Seyfried's work to establish the Glucose Ketone Index (GKI).[108] In other words, dial down the carb intake.

The same applies if you are overweight or have gut issues as a high fat low carb macro ratio will amplify the effects of ketosis and accelerate both fat burning and the repair of your overall microbiome.

1-2 Day Cycle Off (Optional)

You can optionally cycle off high fat, low carb, and low protein macros by lowering fat and boosting carbs and protein 1-2 days per week to provide more flexible eating and according to Dr. Joseph Mercola an extra boost of human growth hormone.

Additionally, by cycling off for 1-2 days you may be able to help preserve insulin sensitivity right after a prolonged (5 day) suppression of insulin during your keto log burning cycle.   And since you want to be able to burn fat, carbs and protein efficiently this could be a power boosting strategy.

Just remember, our ancestors more than likely cycled off burning primarily fat on occasions, like when they found a beehive full of honey or a bounty of berries in the spring or summer.

So if you do choose to cycle off just make sure you aren't binging on cupcakes and steaks but rather slightly boosting your intake 1-2 days a week with nutrient dense foods from the "Power Boost" category.

The following recommendations would be a realistic shift in your macros when you cycle off for a day or two.

✓ Med Fat - 30-50 % of calories from healthy fats
✓ Med Carb - 30-50 % of calories from carbs
✓ Med Protein - 10-30 % of calories from protein

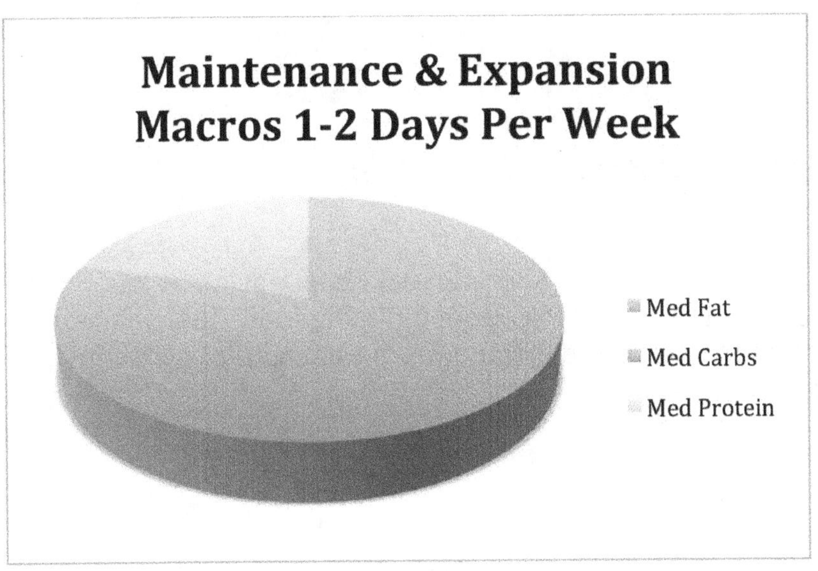

While these ranges are recommendations for optimal health and maximum power, don't worry about getting your macros exact. In fact, if you focus on the quality of your food first and commit to experimenting within these ranges, you'll get close to your sweet spot of maximum power, which is all you'll need to turn the tide and experience amazing results. So remember, **focus on high quality food first!** Second, experiment with quantity!

The High Fat Heroes (50% – 70%)

Now that you understand macros, I'm guessing at this point you want to know more about the tasty foods that will be on your next plate. And since you'll be eating mostly fat, let's start with that.

Fat Is Your Friend

If the title of this section seems at all out of alignment with your beliefs or public opinion, there's a good reason. Over the last several decades dietary fats have been vilified as the cause for a host of diseases including obesity, diabetes and heart disease. This, in turn, has created a low-fat craze never seen before in the history of the world.

Unfortunately, the results have been devastating - the opposite of what one would have expected.

According to the Journal of American Medical Association, almost 4 in 10 American adults over the age of 20 (40%) were considered obese in 2015 and 2016, a sharp increase over the 33.7% who were obese in 2007 and 2008.[109]

Fortunately, the scientific community has debunked most of the pseudoscience surrounding the obesity epidemic and revealed the real culprit – sugar and the overconsumption of carbohydrates.

Nowadays, it's not uncommon to see the addition of healthy fats to restaurant menus and doctors actually recommending the consumption of healthy fat as a prescription for health and weight loss.

But before you dive into a bucket of French fries soaked in a vat of grease fat, you should know the difference between power boosting and power draining fat.

Cooked Fat vs. Raw Fat

If you love frying food in a pan or cooking with oils it's important to understand that overcooking fats can make them rancid and result in oxidative damage, which drains your power.

We mentioned this earlier but it's crucial to start cooking with a steamer or lower the heat as low as possible when you sauté. Remember, overcooked and overheated fat oxidizes and similar to "water that makes iron rusty," makes your joints tendons and skin acidic and brittle.

Additionally, you don't have to cook fat to make it rancid or toxic. For example, nuts will go rancid if they are not eaten within a certain amount of time, regardless of how you store or cook them. How long is widely debated but there is one factor you cannot debate and that is: taste.

If you bite into a nut and it seems extra chewy or doesn't taste good (rubbery, not crunchy with a rancid flavor) there's a very good chance it's rancid and toxic. Here are a few guidelines to make sure you're not eating toxic nuts and oils:

- **Store Nuts In The Refrigerator -** This keeps them fresher longer.
- **Buy Whole Nuts** - Chopped and pieced nuts go rancid much quicker than whole nuts.
- **Buy Sealed Bags** – Don't buy bin nuts as the nuts in bins have been sitting there for a long time exposed to oxygen which means they are oxidized and rotting.
- **Don't Buy Big** – Big bags of nuts or large bottles of oils that take months to consume go rancid. While you may be getting a financial bargain from buying big items, your hospital bill will more than offset any financial savings when you find yourself sick from eating rancid nuts and oils.

The Two Types Of Fat

There are two types of fat, saturated and unsaturated. Choosing which fats to eat is a highly debated issue and requires a little investigation, so let's get clear on what the science says.

Saturated Fats

First off, saturated fats come primarily from animal based sources and include:

1) **Dairy foods** - butter, cream, ice cream, milk and cheese

2) **Meat, Poultry & Eggs** – red meat, poultry and eggs from animals

3) **Plant Products** - coconut (oil, cream, butter), palm oil and cooking margarine

4) **Processed foods** - deep fried foods (e.g. chips, battered foods) packaged cakes, biscuits, pastries and pies.

When people think about eating saturated fat, more often than not, they think about the purported cholesterol clogging effects on your arteries and the potential for heart disease. But according to Harvard Health, most of the cholesterol in your body does not come from food, it comes from your liver.[110]

In reality, cholesterol is simply your body's natural response to patch up the holes burnt into your arteries from all the inflammation created by the overconsumption of sugar and refined carbs.

Of course, this points us to one of the main culprits of all disease, that 4th category above - "Processed foods." And while processed foods should be avoided at all costs, the other three categories above have gotten a bad rap.

If you're at all doubtful of this assertion, you may want to look up a landmark systematic review and meta-analysis of observational studies, which showed no association between saturated fat consumption and all-cause mortality, coronary heart disease, ischemic stroke or type 2 diabetes in healthy adults.[111]

Further bolstering this evidence is another meta-analysis, which pooled data from 21 studies and included nearly 348,000 adults. Remarkably, this study found no difference in the risks of heart disease and stroke between people with the lowest and highest intakes of saturated fat.[112]

In a 1992 editorial published in the Archives of Internal Medicine, Dr. William Castelli, a former director of the Framingham Heart study, stated:

"In Framingham, Mass., the more saturated fat one ate, the more cholesterol one ate, the more calories one ate, the lower the person's serum cholesterol. The opposite of what… Keys et al would predict…We found that the people who ate the most cholesterol, ate the most saturated fat, ate the most calories, weighed the least and were the most physically active."[113]

And if you love eggs, you're going to love this next study, which was published in the International Journal of Obesity. In summary, researchers fed participants either bagels or eggs for breakfast over an 8-week period and found that the egg eaters lost 61% more weight than the bagel eaters.[114]

And finally, the icing on the proverbial cake (hopefully made with coconut oil), revealed quite the opposite of what most would expect when researchers discovered that with every 30-point reduction in cholesterol, mortality (death) increased 22%.[115]

In light of these studies, it's important you understand that cholesterol is a good thing, which you can't live without.

For instance, did you know that roughly 60% of your brain is made of fat and roughly 25% of that is cholesterol? This explains why many people on low-fat diets often feel tired and lose focus - your brain needs fat for both energy and overall maintenance.

But that's not it, cholesterol has a host of power boosting awesomeness including:

- Builds the structure of cell membranes.
- Makes hormones like estrogen, testosterone and adrenal hormones.
- Helps you produce vitamin D and increase the efficiency of your metabolism.
- Protects your heart.

Neu5Gc

While there are clear benefits from eating saturated fats, the real challenge is the byproducts that come primarily from meat, which contains a sugar molecule incompatible with human biochemistry.

In particular, Neu5Gc is a sugar molecule found in beef, lamb and pork, which according to several studies creates inflammation, autoimmune disorders and cancer.[116]

Interestingly, since humans and chickens do not carry the Neu5Gc sugar molecule but instead carry the Neu5Ac molecule, studies show beef eaters have a much higher incidence of cancer than chicken eaters[117]

Advanced Glycation End Products (AGEs)

Adding fuel to the fire on the grill are advanced glycation end products (AGEs), which are harmful compounds formed when protein or fat combine with sugar in your bloodstream.

So if you're cooking on the grill a lot you should know that foods that have been exposed to high temperatures from grilling, frying, or toasting, tend to be very high in these compounds and according to studies can lead to cancer and a host of other illnesses.[118]

The Blue Zones

Lastly, since longevity in my book is synonymous with power, we'll also need to research the longest-lived societies and model the power foods they eat if we are to uncover our own fountain of youth.

In this respect, The Blue Zones, a book written by National Geographic fellow Dan Buettner, is arguably one of the main authorities on the topic.

Interestingly, Dan traveled the world with National Geographic and while documenting the different lifestyles of various cultures discovered that people in certain regions of the world live much longer than average. These long-lived

societies came from five different regions and were dubbed
"The Blue Zones" as follows:

1) Okinawa (Japan)
2) Sardinia (Italy)
3) Nicoya (Costa Rica)
4) Icaria (Greece)
5) Seventh-day Adventists (Loma Linda, California)

Ironically, the one thing in common, which all regions shared was that they all ate a primarily plant based diet with very little animal protein.

While this may be shocking to some, just remember, *The Power Diet* is a flexible diet and allows you to test out new solutions without a massive shock to your system. Accordingly, we'll be including just the right amount of both saturated and unsaturated fats to create maximum power and longevity.

Additionally, I will continue to encourage you to experiment by adding or subtracting power foods to find your own sweet spot of maximum power and… happy taste buds!

Unsaturated Fats

To achieve maximum power we'll be focusing primarily on the two types of unsaturated fats, monounsaturated and polyunsaturated, which studies show lower LDL blood cholesterol. And if you have a history of heart disease or gut issues in the family you'll also be happy to learn multiple studies have shown the consumption of unsaturated fats to be linked with a lower risk of heart disease and better gut health.[119]

Specifically, monounsaturated fats (MUFA) are found in plant foods like avocados, olive oil and nuts, while polyunsaturated fats (PUFA) include omega-3 fatty acids from sources like pastured eggs, oily fish such as salmon, tuna, sardines and anchovies, as well and nuts and seeds like walnuts and flax seeds.

Monounsaturated fats also contain omega-6 fatty acids, which are found in some power draining oils like safflower and canola but can also be found in some power boosters like sesame seeds, hemp seeds and pine nuts.

This is significant since studies show a diet higher in omega-6 as compared to long-chain omega-3 may promote insulin resistance, inflammation, cancer and obesity.[120] And since the typical Western diet contains an unhealthy ratio of 15:1 omega-6 fats to omega-3 fats it's absolutely crucial you familiarize yourself with the biggest power boosters of omega-3 fats and make sure you don't fall into this trap. [121]

Specifically, we'll be shooting for a 3:1 ratio of omega-6 fats vs. omega-3 fats as studies show this to be highly beneficial in lowering inflammation.[122] So for every one gram of omega-3 food, you can eat three grams of omega-6 fats. And remember, according to Dr. Joseph Mercola you should keep your percentage of total calories of omega-6 fats below 4% because they will damage your cellular and mitochondrial membranes.

Since omega-6 fats are so prevalent in nuts, seeds and plants we're going to focus primarily on the omega-3 fats to make the distinction between the two super simple.

As you read my top 10 list of omega-3 power boosters below notice how much of these foods are on your typical plate. (Note: all fish are wild caught)

Omega 3 Power Boosters

1. Salmon
2. Mackerel
3. Trout
4. Walnuts
5. Sardines
6. Anchovies
7. Grass fed beef
8. Grass fed butter
9. Pastured eggs
10. Spirulina

If you're eating "Power Foods" from *The Power Diet* you won't need to worry about getting enough omega-6 foods. What you will need to consciously be aware of is whether or not you're getting enough of these omega-3 fats. Make sure you don't fall short by adding some of these to each meal.

High Fat Hero Options

In order to fill up your plate with enough power boosting fat, you'll need to continue to familiarize yourself with the foods that will dominate your plate. I call these the high fat heroes. And since most people struggle to decipher how many fats vs. carbs vs. proteins are in a particular food I've created two categories to ease this process as follows:

Primary - foods, which contain over 50% of a particular macro. For example, most nuts contain over 50% fat, which makes this their primary category.

Secondary - foods that contain less than 50% of a macro. For example, most nuts contain slightly less than 50% protein, which makes protein their secondary category.

The goal here is to simply get familiar with the primary macros in your foods so you can add or subtract without having to do a lot of calculations. Make a mental note of the following high fat heroes:

Primary – Contains Over 50% Fat

✓ Avocados

✓ Coconut (oil, cream, butter) MCT oil, XCT oil

✓ Raw cacao butter

✓ Grass fed butter, ghee, cream (preferably raw and organic)

✓ Grass fed cheese (preferably raw)

✓ Nuts & Seeds – Blanched almonds, walnuts, pecans, pistachios, macadamia, pine, brazil, chestnuts, flax and hemp seeds.

✓ Oils – Olive, coconut, macadamia, MCT, avocado, perilla, walnut, red palm, rice bran, sesame, cod

Secondary – Contains Under 50% Fat

✓ Fish (low mercury, wild caught) – Sardines, anchovies, salmon (sockeye / king), mackerel, herring, cod, petrale sole

✓ Eggs – Organic, pasture raised

✓ Grass fed meats and poultry

✓ Milk – Full cream cow milk (Type 2 casein) sheep or goat

How Much Fat Will Be On My Plate?

In my experience, most people have no interest in counting calories or breaking out a calculator when deciding how much to eat. This brings us back to "Mindful Eating" which we mentioned earlier.

In the beginning, you'll need to dial in your sweet spot and make a little extra effort by mindfully measuring how many grams per macro are in the food on your plate.

Then, once you get familiar with the visual representation of how much you need to hit your sweet spot of power foods, you can simply eyeball the plate and chow down.

Just remember, when it comes to fat, your plate will contain over 50% healthy fats, which contain twice as many calories as protein and carbs. So when you look at your plate, from a purely visual standpoint, even though the fat may represent 50% in total calories, it will not cover 50% of your plate. Instead, it will cover about half that, which is around 25% or ¼. So remember:

Cover at least ¼ (25%) of your plate with Fat!

And don't worry about getting it exact. You can always remove or add fat depending on your goals and how it makes you feel. For now, shoot for a goal of loading your next plate with at least 25% from the fat sources just mentioned.

Signs You're Eating Too Much Fat

So let's say you're shooting for that 50%-70% fat range but how do you really know if you're eating too much or too little?

Healthy fats help you think, sustain energy and absorb vitamins. Accordingly, an imbalance of consumption results in the breakdown of these processes. Let's talk about the signs of imbalanced fat intake so you can make adjustments and find your sweet spot of optimum power.

If you're eating too much you'll experience some of the symptoms listed below. Keep in mind, if you're dealing with some form of illness or a cold this will only exaggerate the imbalance.

Diarrhea - Unabsorbed fat can cause your small intestines and colon to secrete more water, resulting in what Bulletproof Diet creator Dave Asprey likes to call "disaster pants" (aka Diarrhea). While you could be over consuming healthy fats from *The Power Diet*, most challenges here come from cooked and processed fats, which are highly toxic as mentioned earlier.

Gas & Bloating - If you are lactose intolerant and have a hard time digesting raw or pasteurized dairy you will most likely experience diarrhea, gas, bloating and heartburn. If this is you, eliminate all dairies except for butter and ghee, which has little to no lactose.

Acid Reflux / Heartburn / GERD – While you may have heard that dairy, spicy foods, processed fats, alcohol and in general overly acidic foods can cause heartburn (GERD) it's important to understand that even healthy fats eaten in excess can cause this as well.

I learned this recently by making a super green fat smoothie with 80% fat and drinking it until I was 100% full. Within about 10 minutes I felt the fiery eruption of stomach acid from my gut into my mouth. It was actually quite a shock because I thought I was eating a really healthy smoothie and I hadn't felt heartburn in years.

What I realized was that I was not only eating too much food but my macros were simply too high in fat.

The lesson? Make sure you stick to the recommended macro ranges and always stop eating before you are full (more on this later).

Signs You're Not Eating Enough Fat

If you're not eating enough fat, this could be a little easier to detect since there are some telltale signs of imbalance such as:

Dry Skin, Eyes, Hair and Hair Loss - Healthy fat from *The Power Diet* functions as a lubricant that keeps your skin, hair and eyes lubricated. If you experience dry body parts and cannot attribute it to climate or low water consumption, you may not be eating enough healthy fats.

Constant fatigue - If you lack energy and concentration and cannot attribute it to lack of sleep or overexertion, there's a good chance you need to up your fat intake. One of the biggest telltale signs of under consumption of fat is during your fasting period. If you skip breakfast and your body freaks out, you are most likely not yet metabolically flexible or simply not eating enough fat.

In the case of the former, you may just need to continue following the guidelines of The Power Diet especially the last chapter "Frequency."

Never Feeling Full, Constant Hunger - If you need to snack often, again, you have yet to become fat adapted (metabolically flexible) and are more than likely dependent on carbohydrates as your main fuel source. If this is you just follow *The Power Diet* protocol and soon enough you'll cut the chains of carboholic syndrome.

Hormonal Problems, Highly Irritable – First off, it's important to understand that hormones are formed from fat and cholesterol; without them, hormone production would fall apart and so would you.

For example, women who don't eat enough healthy fat may experience the loss of their menstrual cycle when they should normally be getting it. Fats also help you absorb fat-soluble vitamins like A, D, E and K and a deficiency in any of these can cause a hormonal imbalance, and turn you into a train wreck nobody wants to be around.

Stick To *The Power Diet* Protocol

If you feel any of these symptoms and you are not suffering from some other illness you can simply add or subtract fat depending on your circumstances and test it for 30 days. If you feel improvement, continue doing what you're doing, and if not, you may just need to adjust your other macros (carbs and protein).

Now let's recap what we know about power draining, power limiting and power boosting fats.

✓ **Power Drain:** Overly cooked fats and oils, deep fried foods (e.g. chips, battered foods) packaged cakes, biscuits, pastries and pies.
✓ **Power Limit:** Too many saturated fats like meat, poultry and dairy (limit these to 1-3 days a week)
✓ **Power Boost:** Raw fat, grass fed butter, unsaturated fats like fish, avocados, nuts, seeds and oils

The Carbo Kings (10% - 30%)

Earlier we learned about the potential to fall into the carboholic trap by eating too many carbs, especially the refined variety, like candies, cookies, donuts, potato chips, and crackers.

Unfortunately, eating these is like throwing match sticks on your campfire, eventually, your glucose levels in your bloodstream elevate insulin levels beyond healthy limits, at which point glucose gets stored as fat. And this doesn't even account for the extra surge of cortisol from burning match sticks all the time.

Yes, sadly, eating refined carbs or too many carbs in general, jacks up your cortisol levels, which can put you in a state of fight or flight, create more inflammation and keep you up all night.[123] [124]

And for those that struggle with excess weight issues, you'll want to shoot for the lower end of the recommended carbohydrate range by eating closer to 10% of your total calories as carbs.

To boost power in this department we're going to minimize our carb intake and eliminate the refined carbs altogether. But again, don't worry; this is not an extreme carbohydrate elimination diet. You need carbohydrates for fuel and in some cases to fight off a virus.

Feed A Virus – Starve A Bacterium

You may have heard the old rephrase "Feed a fever and starve a cold," but what you may not have heard is the recommendation to feed a virus carbs and starve a bacterial infection from those same carbs. As odd as this may sound, according to a National Institute of Health funded research team, this may have real implications for killing viruses and bacterial infections that make you ill.

In this study, researchers found that mice infected with the influenza virus significantly improved their survival when fed glucose, while the exact opposite proved true in mice infected with *Listeria*, a fever-inducing bacterium. According to the study:

"When researchers forced Listeria-infected mice to consume even a small amount of food, they all died." [125]

So what does this mean for you?

Essentially by starving a harmful bacterium like Listeria, you starve them from their own food source and they die off. And while you will not want to starve off a harmful virus like you would a bacterium, by sticking to the recommendations of *The Power Diet* you can have your cake and eat it too.

So for example, if you contract a virus you could move your carbohydrate intake closer to the upper recommended limits with a potential additional increase of another 5%, which would bring your total carb intake per day to 25-30% of total macros.

In contrast, if you have a bacterial infection you can reduce your carb intake to the lower recommended limits with a potential subtraction of another 5%, which would bring your total carb intake per day to 5-10% of total macros.

Just keep in mind, not all carbohydrates are equal. So while you'll want to stay in those recommended ranges, you'll also want to stick to the recommended "Power Foods" of *The Power Diet*.

And now that you're armed with some pathogen protection power, let's take a look at the power boosting carbs that will be on your next plate of food.

Vegetables

Loaded with powerful antioxidants, vitamins, minerals and phytochemicals that keep you young, powerful and vibrant, veggies will take up a majority of your plate and help you maintain your 3:1 alkaline ratio balance.

The primary macro for plants is carbohydrates and is more often than not concentrated in the fiber, which does not get digested as sugar but instead functions as food for your good bacteria as well as a broom to sweep out unwanted invaders.

In *The Power Diet,* we'll be getting our carbs primarily from vegetables and starches, both raw and lightly cooked.

Prebiotic Veggies

As a reoccurring theme in The Power Diet, taking care of your microbiome will be a major factor when it comes time to select vegetables that provide maximum power.   In this respect, no significant result could be achieved without addressing both probiotics and prebiotics.

In a nutshell, while "Probiotics" produce beneficial bacteria with specialized supplements and foods like yogurt, raw butter, and sauerkraut, "Prebiotics" provide food for those "Probiotics."

Later on, we'll talk about supplementing with both probiotics and prebiotics but I recommend getting most of these from foods. So while *The Power Diet* includes power veggies like broccoli, cauliflower and lettuces, which all function as prebiotics to a certain degree, we'll also be focusing on high powered veggies that contain the highest proportions of prebiotics like jicama, dandelion greens, arugula, asparagus, leeks, sweet potatoes, yams, green bananas and watermelon radish.

One of the primary substances found in these foods is called inulin, a prebiotic fiber that nourishes your gut bacteria, helps manage weight, and improves digestion, immunity and heart health.[126] [127] [128]

To capitalize on the power of prebiotics we'll be adding in healthy doses of both vegetables and starches that contain inulin.

Dairy

With the exception of butter and cheese, which are primarily fat, dairy such as milk and yogurt are comprised mostly of carbohydrates.

As mentioned earlier, pasteurization kills off vital enzymes and nutrients so if you do choose to eat dairy and you don't have any negative reactions I highly recommend buying "raw" varieties if at all possible.

As a second level of caution for dairy lovers, you'll also need to consider the problem of grain and soy fed dairy, which can be problematic due to reactive lectins. Make sure you purchase "Type 2" casein dairy products, which do not contain reactive lectins like Type 1 casein.

Alternatively, you can choose grass fed dairy products from sheep or goats, which have little to no casein and are more easily digested.

Let's go ahead and check out the primary and secondary sources of carbohydrates, which will fill up a majority of your plate.

Carbo King Options

Primary – Contains Over 50% Carbs

- ✓ Starches – Sweet potato, yam and carrots. Shirataki or kelp noodles. Green bananas, green papaya, Roots and Tubers including Jerusalem artichoke, taro, beets, chicory, yakon, konjac, parsnip, rutabaga and turnip.

- ✓ Power Vegetables – Broccoli, cauliflower, arugula, spinach, kale, chard, collards, romaine, butter leaf, red leaf, kale, cabbage, chicory root, radish, celery, bok choy.

- ✓ Pre-Biotic Veggies - Fennel, jicama, garlic, onions, leeks, cabbage, dandelion greens, radishes, artichoke, asparagus, and parsley.

- ✓ Legumes, lentils and beans, which have been pressure cooked and/or sprouted, and soaked.

- ✓ Grains & Grain Substitutes - White rice, millet, and sourdough. Flours including: almond, coconut, cassava, pecan, walnut, tapioca, arrowroot & acacia.

✓ Fruits (low sugar) – berries when in season

✓ Dairy – Grass fed (preferably raw), type 2 casein milk and yogurt from cows, goat or sheep milk and yogurt.

Secondary – Contains Under 50% Carbs

✓ Nuts & Seeds – Almonds (blanched), walnuts, pecans, pistachios, macadamia, pine, flax, hemp, brazil, chestnut

How Many Carbs Will Be On My Plate?

Carbs from *The Power Diet* are loaded with fiber, which is not as dense as fat or protein so they will take up a majority of your plate.

For example, from a purely visual standpoint, a serving of veggies on *The Power Diet* will take up roughly 40–50% of your plate and a serving of starches will fill up roughly 10-20%, which brings us to 50-70%. Keep in mind; this is not the total calorie percentage but simply a visual representation.

Again, you can adjust these serving sizes according to your goals and how they make you feel but to get started shoot for a goal of loading your next plate with a majority (at least 60%) from the sources just mentioned.

**Cover the majority of your plate with healthy carbs!
(40-50% veggies & 10-20% starches)**

Signs You're Eating Too Many Carbs

Power veggies and starches are clearly good for us but like anything else, eating too much can backfire. So how do you know if you're eating too many carbs?

Essentially, when you eat carbs they are broken down and turned into glucose much more quickly than protein and fat, which you'll most likely feel as a rush of energy from that feel good hormone we mentioned earlier - serotonin.

At this point, you'll feel a jolt of energy, like you need to stand up and move your body. This is the sugar high we see when kids (sometimes adults) eat candy.

They explode with energy but it's short lived and ends in agitation, lack of focus and a need for more speed (more carbs). If this is you, pay attention, this is your first sign you have too many carbs in your diet and it's time to dial it back.

But you don't need to eliminate carbs. As we mentioned earlier you need the good carbs from *The Power Diet*.

The Sugar Crash
This problem occurs when there is not enough fat, fiber or protein to slow down the glucose from carbs that enter your bloodstream and sustain your energy. And as quickly as you can jumpstart your mood from a shot of coca cola or a dose of potato chips, once you stop eating those carbs, your blood sugar and good mood will plummet like a drop down a steep rollercoaster - into a dungeon of depression.

At this point, you'll more than likely feel the infamous "sugar crash" that overconsumption of carbs invariably delivers.   If this happens, make sure you dial it back and reduce if not eliminate those carbs.

Carbo Cravings
When the sugar crash happens you may feel an insatiable desire to continue stuffing more of those carbs (potato chips, crackers, soda, juice, fruit, candy, etc.) down your throat or artificially inflate your energy with a caffeinated beverage or mind-altering drug. This is the second signal you are eating too many carbs – dial it back!

You Can't Lose Weight
If you find losing weight extra challenging, you'll need to back off on the carbs. We mentioned this earlier but it's important you shoot for the lower range of carb consumption as roughly 10% of your total macros. Essentially, to expedite your weight loss you'll need to cut out 10-20% of

the carbs you're consuming and employ the use of an optimized fitness program like <u>Fired Up</u>.

Tired and Unproductive
Yes, it gets worse. If you continue to feed yourself more of that carbo crack or jack yourself up with too much caffeine crack you'll also more than likely feel your energy plummet and become highly incompetent, unproductive or just fall asleep at a time when you would normally be awake.

This is your third signal you're eating too many carbs. Make sure you look for these signals and lower your carb intake if you feel the following:

- A jolt of energy that is unsustainable and ends in a crash.

- An insatiable desire to continue eating more carbs or drink a caffeinated beverage.

- Lack of energy, unproductive or sleeping at an odd time.

In contrast, while the carboholic cycle may feel like a horrible old broken rollercoaster, eating healthy fat is a much more sustainable source of energy simply because it burns fuel at a much slower rate over a longer period of time. This, of course, is highly significant since jacking up your carb intake jacks up your insulin and throws your hormones and your mood way out of balance.

Signs You're Not Eating Enough Carbs

In many Ketogenic diets, the carbohydrates are highly restricted; some as little as 5% of total calories, which myself and many other experts believe is not a good long-term strategy.

In contrast, *The Power Diet* offers plenty of room for healthy carbohydrates with plenty of fiber and doesn't have any of the negative side effects of these highly restrictive ketogenic diets.

That being said, you should know what signs to look for, if in fact, you need to boost your carb intake into the upper recommended ranges in order to increase your power.

Feeling Weak

The main thing to look for here is a lack of energy and poor concentration. For example, if you feel really weak during exercise, this could be an indication of an inability to burn fat as fuel (not yet metabolically flexible) or just not enough carbs in your diet.

Yes, this sign is identical to the sign from eating too many carbs but there is a big difference here.

In this case, if you have already gone through the phase of becoming metabolically flexible and you feel low on energy and can't concentrate, you'll need to ask yourself two questions:

1) Did I get an unsustainable jolt of energy from the last food or drink I consumed?

2) Do I feel an insatiable desire to eat carbs because I just recently put down a bag of chips, soda or other high carb food?

If the answer to these two questions is "No" then you need to boost your carb intake. And if you're uncertain how to become metabolically flexible and start burning more fat without the cravings for carbs, don't worry, because our next chapter is going to turn you into a lean mean fat burning machine.

Before we do that, let's recap what we know about the power draining, power limiting and power boosting carbs from *The Power Diet*.

✓ **Power Drain:** whole grains, beans, toxic lectin veggies and starches, high sugar fruits
✓ **Power Limit:** white rice, millet, fermented sourdough, garlic, raw beets, collards, kale, chard and spinach. Peeled, deseeded & cooked pumpkin, squash & zucchini. Sprouted, soaked, fermented and/or pressure cooked legumes, beans, lentils and quinoa.
✓ **Power Boost:** low lectin veggies and starches, grain substitutes, limited low sugar fruits, dairy and nuts.

The Protein Powerhouses (10% - 20%)

While nobody disputes the power and essential nature of protein in building muscles, how much and what type has been a highly debated and misunderstood topic with no shortage of opinionated experts. Accordingly, we'll be kicking off the protein powerhouses by first addressing the "how much" question.

While certain individuals may have a larger requirement for protein than a normal person (elderly, athletes and highly active people), studies show the first big problem with this macro comes from simply eating too much of it. [129] [130]

For example, the average American eats twice as much protein as they need, which leads to weight gain and a massive drain in power. [131]

In a landmark study from the American Dietetic Association, researchers fed 30 grams of protein to one group and 90 grams to anther. Remarkably, the researchers found that there was no additional benefit to eating more than 30 grams of protein in one meal. [132]

Of course, this begs the question: "What happened to the other 60 grams of protein that did not go through the process of protein synthesis and turn into muscle?"

In a process known as glycogenesis, the extra protein from overconsumption was turned into fat. Obviously, this is not good news if you're overweight or trying to stay lean and powerful.

Protein Increases Insulin

Similar to carbohydrates, the overconsumption of protein also leads to an overabundance of glucose with a resulting insulin spike and an inflammation bomb. Perhaps you can remember a time you felt this bomb drop. If not, you can test it out by simply eating a big steak or a bucket of chicken.

What you'll notice is a massive spike of energy, with a resulting crash that will most likely leave you on the sidelines, perhaps asleep drooling on the couch with the TV on. Not exactly the vision of powerful we're looking for.

You're Body Supplies Protein From Within

Perhaps even more revealing about any overconsumption of protein is the fact that we humans recycle approximately 20 grams of our own protein every day.[133] And according to Dr. Steven Gundry,

"Protein that has been shed from your intestines and mucus gets recycled. So, when mucus gets made, or the cells that make up your gut lining die and are replaced, you digest the proteins."

So while you may think you need a big steak or boatload of protein to be powerful, you're already getting extra protein you don't even know about. So on top of the exorbitant amounts recommended by so-called nutrition experts, it's highly likely you're draining your power by eating too much.

Calorie Restriction Leaves Clues

If you're not yet on board with the reduction of protein, please allow me to throw a few more smart bombs on the grill.

This story starts with one of the most unpleasant diets in the world, the calorie restriction diet. To be clear, while *The Power Diet* will restrict calories at certain times during the day, it's not an extreme calorie restriction diet that makes you starve from hunger and feel deprived.

The point here is to simply observe the effects of reducing protein in caloric restriction studies and how this can increase your lifespan. In this regard, a significant increase in lifespan has been observed in several animal studies and there is now evidence that this same benefit occurs in humans.[134] [135] [136]

What's most interesting is that current research shows that it's not the restriction of total calories that triggers the beneficial effects of calorie-restricted diets. Instead, the latest science suggests that this phenomenon may actually be the result of simply lowering your protein intake – most importantly your meat consumption, which contains high levels of the amino acid methionine.[137]

Insulin Overwhelm

We talked about insulin in The Carbo Kings but it also applies to protein and because it's so crucial to your power or lack thereof we're going to investigate just a little further.

Insulin is a hormone made by your pancreas that allows your body to use sugar (glucose) from carbohydrates and protein in the food you eat for energy or to store for later use during times of scarcity. It's also a regulating mechanism that helps keep your blood sugar level from getting too high (hyperglycemia) or too low (hypoglycemia).

What's important to understand about insulin is that eating excess protein and carbs increases insulin, makes you less sensitive to insulin and throws another bomb on the grill.

Since studies of both healthy humans and centenarians (people who live over 100) have been shown to have lower than average insulin levels and greater insulin receptor sensitivity *The Power Diet* protocol aims to model this longevity strategy by lowering both your protein and carbohydrate consumption to more healthy levels.[138]

TMAO Trouble

We'll talk about those recommended levels shortly. For now, we have two more really important bombs to dodge, the first of which is TMAO (trimethylamine N-oxide).

As a well-known inflammatory molecule derived from meat and other animal products, TMAO can compromise the health of your microbiome in a big way.[139]

For example, just by eating a single hamburger, studies have shown TMAO to drop a virtual bomb in your gut by increasing inflammation up to 70%, while at the same time impairing blood flow throughout your entire body.[140]

We've talked a lot about inflammation and it's connection to diseases like cancer and heart disease and now it's time to face the music by dialing down the consumption of animal products.   You can still eat these occasionally but if you really want to maximize your power and longevity they should be reduced to 1-3 times per week or as a treat once in a while.

mTOR Monster

If those bombs don't scare you straight and dial down your protein dosage, maybe the monster "mTOR" will.

As the key muscle-building mechanism in all mammals, mTOR was discovered by scientists when looking for a solution to cancer.

What's important to understand about this ancient protein is that excess protein consumption activates it and virtually all cancers are associated with mTOR activation. Thus, the prevention of mTOR with drugs, such as rapamycin, for which mTOR is named, is one of the most common and highly effective anticancer treatments today.

Fortunately, when mTOR is turned off, it instructs your body's cells to fire up repair and maintenance processes like autophagy (more on this later), DNA repair, and activation of intracellular antioxidants. According to Dr. Joseph Mercola, when you eat too much protein:

"It cues the cell to grow and proliferate; it also suppresses most cellular and mitochondrial repair and regeneration mechanisms. If you maintain low levels of glucose, excess amino acids, insulin, and growth factors (like IGF-1), you will inhibit mTOR, thereby allowing the up-regulation of gene expression that promotes cellular and mitochondrial maintenance and repair."

Further clarifying this need to reduce protein is a pioneer of anti-aging and metabolic medicine Dr. Ron Rosedale who declares:

"As we get older, excessive protein causes the cell to turn a blind eye to aging. But limiting it triggers a beautifully orchestrated network of internal processes that wards off disease, stretching out life and increasing the probability of exercising nature's imperative to reproduce."

Clearly, with all those bombs dropped on overconsumption of protein it's crucial we become extra vigilant on staying within a healthy range that sustains overall energy, power and longevity.

What Is The Best Type Of Protein?

Naturally, this brings us to our next riddle, "what type of protein is best?

If you're thinking about a brawl between carnivores and vegetarians, think again. We're not interested in who's right or wrong here, we're only interested in truth and power. And when it comes to power no truth would be complete without a reality check on amino acids.

How Do I Get My Aminos?

While it's no mystery that animal sources of protein contain all of the vital amino acids for building muscle, one of the biggest myths surrounding plant based vegetable sources is that they do not.

Sorry to drop another bomb here but since truth is our most potent destroyer of ignorance I'm going to let you in on one of the largest studies ever undertaken, which compared the nutrient intake of meat-eaters vs. plant-eaters. Can you guess the results?

Researchers concluded that the average plant-eater not only gets enough protein but consumes 70% more than they need. [141]

As for those amino acids, the science here is also indisputable and shows us that all plants contain all of the essential amino acids. [142] [143] [144]

If you're short on examples look no further than the powerhouse spirulina, a blue-green algae that is roughly 60% protein. For example, my favorite organic, raw recommendation from <u>BN Labs</u> delivers a whopping 8 grams of complete protein in one tablespoon.

But that's not it, spirulina from <u>BN Labs</u> also delivers 16% of your daily requirements for iron and thiamin and 400% of your daily vitamin A needs along with a healthy dose of the all-important omega-3 fatty acids we talked about earlier. [145]

But perhaps the most crucial power boost of all comes from its delivery of 163% of your daily requirement for vitamin B-12. So if you're not eating animal or fish sources to meet your protein macro requirement this is absolutely crucial since lack of B-12 is tied to lack of energy, focus and a host of illnesses including Crohn's, celiac, anemia, graves and lupus.[146]

Since vitamin B-12 is rarely found in the plant world, superfoods like spirulina become even more crucial when dialing down your consumption of animal based protein. And considering it has one of the highest measurements of megahertz energy (170) I recommend adding this in as a replacement for animal protein 2-4 days a week.

It's also important to note that even though some plant foods are lower in certain amino acids than others when you consume plants your body breaks down protein into individual amino acids so that the appropriate proteins can be assembled when you need them.

And here's the coconut icing on the primarily plant based diet: If you're using both *The Power Diet* and *Fired Up* to gain maximum power, strength and muscle, research repeatedly demonstrates that as long as you're eating the right amount of amino acids, the source is irrelevant.[147]

For these and other reasons mentioned throughout this book, we'll be focusing on boosting plant-based proteins and limiting your animal based protein.

But again, this is a flexible diet that allows you to experiment and find your own personal sweet spot. For some, this may mean limiting animal based protein and for others, it may mean eliminating them altogether. Make sure you stay open to experimentation and let go of any attachments to an outcome.

And now that you're properly educated on the facts of protein let's go ahead and take a look at the protein powerhouses that should fill up 10-20% of your plate?

Protein Powerhouse Options

Primary – Contains Over 50% Protein

- ✓ Meat and poultry (organic, grass fed and free range)

- ✓ Fish (wild caught, low mercury)

- ✓ Spirulina (organic)

- ✓ Tempeh (grain free organic fermented soy)

- ✓ Hemp tofu (organic grain free)

Secondary – Contains Under 50% Protein

- ✓ Legumes, lentils and beans, (sprouted, soaked and pressure-cooked)

- ✓ Nuts & Seeds – almonds (blanched), walnuts, pecans, pistachios, macadamia, pine, flax, hemp, brazil, chestnut

- ✓ Dairy – Goat, Sheep and Cow (type 2 casein) milk, yogurt, cheese and cream.

- ✓ Vegetables – Broccoli, cauliflower, arugula, spinach, kale, chard, artichoke, asparagus.

How Much Protein Will Be On My Plate?

Since the overconsumption of protein has shown to be a major challenge for most, we'll be mindfully measuring our intake by doing some simple calculations before we start using the eyeball method to find our sweet spot.

To make sure you avoid the trap of mindlessly overeating protein and throwing bombs on yourself, right now we're going to take some action and find just the right amount of protein for your sweet spot of optimum power.

Take Action – Calculate Your Optimal Protein Intake

Because this formula takes into account your ideal body weight, you'll first need to take a quick step back and ask yourself another crucial question:

What Is My Ideal Body Weight?

While *The Power Diet* will help you move towards your ideal weight by simply following its recommendations, by identifying your ideal weight first, you can use this calculation to expedite your journey to maximum power much quicker. As such, you'll need to take action here and identify your ideal weight.

To determine if you are at the proper weight is more intuition than science, so we'll need to investigate a little further with an additional question as follows:

When Did You Last Feel You Were At Your Ideal Weight?

For many people, the answer to this question was high school or college when you were more active. If we think about this logically, unless you're pregnant or training to be a bodybuilder or professional athlete, there is no healthy reason to gain more weight after you've filled out your frame and stopped growing in height.

Even if you've been overweight your whole life I'd wager you probably have a desired weight that you would like to be at. With this in mind you'll need to answer the next question:

What Is My Ideal Weight?

If you don't know just take a guess. Got it? Good, hang on to that number because we'll be using it shortly.

As for science, one of the standard measurements of correct weight is your BMI or Body Mass Index.

Health practitioners use BMI to estimate body fat and possible health risks related to weight. This is important, especially if you've struggled with being overweight and you don't know what your ideal weight is.

To calculate your BMI and ideal weight literally takes 30 seconds, so go ahead and follow the link below and come right back once you find out.

https://chadscottcoaching.com/bmi

Factor In Your Body Type

Question: Did your BMI fall between 18.5 and 24.9? According to the National Heart, Lung and Blood Institute, this is considered a healthy range for ideal body weight. Unfortunately, it's not an exact science, as it does not take into consideration your body type. To get more accurate let's check out the three basic body types and their ideal BMI as follows:

Ectomorphic - Long, lean and thin defines the Ectomorphic body type. If this is you, you most likely have trouble putting muscle on your small frame and have challenges gaining weight, no matter how much you eat. When measuring your BMI your ideal weight should fall in the lower ranges closer to 18.5.

Endomorphic – This body type is the opposite of an Ectomorph and typically possesses larger bones with a fuller figure. If this is you, you'll most likely gain weight easily, have a large bone structure and experience challenges creating muscle definition. When measuring your BMI your ideal weight should fall in the upper ranges around that 24.9 mark.

Mesomorphic – If this is you, you're in the middle and will tend to gain muscle fairly easily. When following good nutrition and exercise, you'll usually have wide shoulders, a small waist, a medium bone structure and low body fat. When measuring your BMI your ideal weight should fall in the mid range around 21.

The 3 Programs

After you've determined your ideal weight, you'll need to pick one of three following routines based on whether or not you're overweight, underweight or at your ideal weight.

Fat Loss (Cutting Phase) 12-Week Program

If you are overweight by more than 10 pounds I recommend focusing on the "Cutting" phase first, which will place a heavy focus on burning off excess fat to restore your body's natural healing powers and restore your mind and body to full power.

As mentioned previously, the quickest way to do this is to follow the recommendations from *The Power Diet* and *Fired Up* programs and shoot for the low-end range for carb consumption (around 10% of daily calories). In most cases, this will translate into reducing your overall carb intake by 10-20% during the course of a day. So if you need to lose weight remember this:

Reduce your carb intake by 10-20%!

Once you do this you should get pretty close to your ideal weight within 8-12-weeks; if not, just keep going until you do. Once you achieve your ideal weight go ahead and switch to "Maintenance & Expansion."

Weight Gain (Bulking) 12-Week Program

If you are underweight and need more bulk I recommend the "Bulking" phase, which will focus on minimizing fat gain with the *Fired Up* program and by upping your carb intake. Keep in mind, this is not a license to become a carboholic. This just means you can shoot for the upper range of carb consumption per day (20% to 30% of daily calories).

Shoot for 20% to 30% carbs per day!

Once you achieve your ideal weight on this program go ahead and switch to the "Maintenance & Expansion" program.

Maintenance & Expansion (M&E)

This program is designed as the ultimate goal of *The Power Diet* and the *Fired Up* program. To be clear, this is not a stagnant (stay the same) routine. Rather, this is a lifestyle change, which will continue to create optimal health and maximum power for the rest of your life.

Once you're at your ideal weight you'll have the flexibility to eat anywhere within *The Power Diet* macro ranges depending on your goals and how you feel.

Can I Lose Weight on Maintenance & Expansion?

I often get asked this question from clients who don't want to cut carbs and increase their fitness routine. The short answer is "Yes" you can lose weight by following the Maintenance and Expansion program. The only difference is that Maintenance & Expansion will simply take longer to lose weight than the cutting program. So if you're ok with potentially doubling the time it takes to get to your ideal weight, then by all means, skip the Fat Loss program and start with Maintenance & Expansion.

How Much Protein Do I Need?

Now that you have a better idea of what your ideal weight should be and which program you're shooting for, it's time to find out how much protein you need.

While this is another widely debated topic, fortunately, we'll be using the science and wisdom of some serious heavyweights in the health and nutrition world including best selling author and founder of the Center For Restorative Medicine, Dr. Steven Gundry and Dr. Valter Longo from The Longevity Institute at the University of Southern California. We'll also back up these two heavyweights with the Food and Nutrition Board of the Institute of Medicine.

And since your age and activity level greatly influence the amount of protein you need we'll also be referencing Dr. Cate Shanahan who created the PRO Nutrition program for the LA Lakers and helped forge a partnership between Whole Foods Market and numerous NBA teams.

It turns out our panel of experts recommend roughly .37 grams of protein per pound of body weight per day for the average sedentary person, so we'll start with this as a base assumption. This .37 represents your **protein variable** and can be changed depending on various circumstances. Let's take a look and an example.

Using a 160-pound person with normal activity level as a hypothetical example, the daily protein requirement would be as follows:

Normal Activity
160 pounds x .37 = 60 Grams or 2.1 Ounces

Since there are 28.4 grams per ounce, a 160-pound person would need 60 grams or slightly over 2 ounces of protein per day. These measurements come in handy when reading labels, as grams don't always appear on packaging.

What If I'm Over 65

If you are over 65 your ability to process protein efficiently will start to decline and you may need more of it to maintain muscle mass, strength and bone health.

In a recent study that followed more than 2,900 seniors over 23 years, researchers found that those who ate the most protein were 30 percent less likely to become functionally impaired than those who ate the least amount.[148]

Accordingly, if you're over 65 you'll need to increase your protein variable to a range of roughly .4 to .5.

What If I'm An Athlete or Highly Active Person?

If you're an athlete or just highly active and burn a lot of calories by working out or exercising you will need even more protein since you will be breaking down more muscle tissue.

The Academy of Nutrition and Dietetics, Dietitians of Canada and the American College of Sports Medicine recommend a protein variable range of roughly .55 to .91 grams per pound of body weight (1.2 - 2 g per kg) per day for athletes, depending on training.[149]

Multiply Your Ideal Weight X Your Protein Variable

In order to determine how much protein per day you need simply multiply your "ideal weight" times your protein variable that seems appropriate for your age and activity level.

For example, if you weigh 161 pounds and you're active or over 65 your total intake of protein per day would look something like the following:

160 pounds x .45 = 72 Grams or 2.6 Ounces

To simplify this process I've created a chart called *The Power Diet Protein Matrix* below. As you can see I've used a protein variable of .37 for normal activity folks, .45 for active or elderly people and .7 for athletes.

The Power Diet Protein Matrix

Ideal Weight	Sedentary Protein Var.37	Active or Elderly Protein Var.45	Athlete Protein Var.7
100-120	37-44	45-54	70-84
121-140	45-52	55-63	85-98
141-160	52-59	64-72	99-113
161-180	60-67	73-81	114-128
181-200	67-74	82-90	129-143
201-220	74-81	91-99	144-158
221-240	82-89	100-108	159-173
241-260	89-96	109-117	174-188
261-280	96-103	118-126	189-203

How To Know For Sure You're Eating Enough Protein

While you can use these average protein variables and multiply them times your ideal weight to find a daily protein requirement, I highly recommend you experiment by significantly dialing down your protein variable by .2 for 10 days then dialing it up .2 for an additional 10 days.

For example, if I'm 160 pounds and active I can experiment for 10 days with 40 grams of protein per day as follows:

160 pounds x .25 = 40 Grams or 1.4 Ounces

For the following 10 days, I would eat 104 grams of protein per day as follows.

160 pounds x .65 = 104 Grams or 3.7 Ounces

If you experiment like this, I can pretty much guarantee you'll notice some striking differences in your overall energy and power.

Once it's clear something is not working, you can simply add or subtract from your protein variable to find your sweet spot. So remember:

**Experiment with your protein variable
until you find your sweet spot!**

What Does A Serving Of Protein Look Like?

While eyeballing your fats and carbs might be relatively simple, when it comes to proteins it can be a little more tricky since protein is dense and more often than not contains fats, proteins and carbs. So again we will return to the importance of mindful eating.

Now that you know how crucial it is to get the right quantity, it's important you spend a few minutes mindfully familiarizing yourself with the amount of grams and ounces typically associated with common portions of power boosting proteins.

In addition, you'll need to start being more mindful about reading labels. We mentioned this previously, but it really makes things simple; and you'll only have to do it for the first month, at which point you'll have memorized your sweet spot for perfect portions.

Below I've listed both Animal and Plant Based protein examples but again, you'll need to use the formulas from above to calculate just how much protein is ideal for you.

WARNING: Overconsumption Of Protein Kills Power!

At this point, I need to issue a second warning. If you do not take into account all sources of protein that go into your meal, chances are you'll end up struggling to dig yourself out of a deep and painful hole from all those bombs mentioned earlier. So in addition to your main protein, whether that's animal or plant based, you will need to factor in all other protein sources including:

- Recycled Protein
- Animal or Fish Sources
- Veggies and Starches
- Nuts and Seeds

If this sounds perplexing, don't worry. Shortly we'll break down most of the key power foods so you can start to familiarize yourself with just how much carbs, fats and protein there are in the foods you'll be eating. But before we do that, we first need to get really clear about the signs of mindless protein intake.

Signs You're Eating Too Much Protein

We talked about the signs of imbalanced consumption from fats and carbs but what about protein? How do you know for sure you're getting too much or not enough?

Most research indicates that eating more than .9 grams per pound of body weight (2 g per kg) daily of protein for a long time can cause health problems.[150] Besides the big crushers like cardiovascular disease, blood vessel disorders, liver and kidney injuries, seizures and death there are some other obvious and not so obvious signs of overconsumption you should pay attention to.

Bad Breath
If you find you have bad breath and it doesn't go away by brushing your teeth and tongue this could be the residue from burning ketones too long. If this is you, dial back your protein and stick to *The Power Diet* recommendations.

Joint Pain
Researchers have found that diets high in red meats can increase the level of uric acid in your blood, which in turn forms painful crystals inside your joints and increases the risk of autoimmune disorders like gout and arthritis.[151]

Dehydration
Ever notice how people (maybe even yourself) need to drink lots of liquid during a meal to get it down the pipes and into the stomach?

One of the primary reasons for this is simply because your body requires water to break down protein and protein (especially cooked protein) doesn't have much water in it. And since your protein doesn't have water as vegetables do, your kidneys, which break down protein, will pull water from elsewhere in your body and leave you dehydrated.

In fact, studies have linked the overconsumption of red meat to kidney disease and shown that as athletes increased their protein consumption they became more dehydrated.[152]

Headaches
As a well-known side effect of dehydration, headaches can be a clear sign you're eating too much protein. Notice if you get headaches shortly after you eat and if so, you'll need to dial it down and check back in with the recommendations from *The Power Diet*.

Constipation
Unfortunately, when you eat too much protein there's also a good chance you're sacrificing the veggies and not getting enough of the fantastic fiber. This will result in constipation and some not so smooth moves. If you're not regular every day, (barring any weird illness) I can guarantee one thing: you're definitely not following the recommendations of *The Power Diet.*

Feeling Weak, Tired and Slow
If you're feeling weak, tired or slow, there's a good chance you're simply eating too much protein. Since protein is much harder to digest than carbs, your body will be overtaxed when you eat too much of it – dial it back.

Now let's review our protein power drains, limits and boosts.

- ✓ **Power Drain:** Grain and/or soy fed meat, poultry and fish. Farmed seafood. Pea, soy, corn or wheat based protein. Packaged meats with preservatives (nitrates, nitrites, sulfates).

- ✓ **Power Limit:** Grass fed or pastured meat & poultry, grass fed whey isolate, factory farmed eggs, shellfish, big fish with high mercury content like tuna, halibut, shark and swordfish.

- ✓ **Power Boost:** Wild caught low mercury fish like sockeye salmon, sardines, petrale sole, anchovies, and arctic cod. Spirulina, nuts and power veggies, hemp tofu, & grain free tempeh.

Stop Guessing And Start Feeling Amazing!

In my experience, most people (I've been guilty) simply pull out food from the refrigerator and mindlessly guess what foods and what quantities would make a great meal.

For instance, most people have no idea when they are eating twice as much protein and half the fat that they need for maximum power. It's no wonder we suffer from all the bombs, power drains and illnesses mentioned earlier.

While we won't be counting calories, in order to really dial in *The Power Diet* and activate maximum power, you'll need to get familiar with the amount of fat, carbs and proteins in your food.

If you're thinking "Oh no, not me, I don't have the time," relax and take a deep breath, because I'm going to make this really simple.

First off, I'm going break down many of the power foods here in this book and second, I've also created an entire video library of step-by-step instructions on how to make 10 minute mouth watering meals that taste rich, savory and delicious.

Once you familiarize yourself with the breakdown of carbs, fats, and proteins in your food and know where your sweet spot is, you won't have to do this ever again for the rest of your life.

Take Action

To help you avoid mindless food preparation that leads to power drain I've created the following Master Mantra for you to remember:

Each time I eat, I am mindful of my macros!

Now go ahead and repeat that mantra 5 times and remember this each time you prepare or order a meal.

To highlight just how important this is, just imagine that a virulent virus rolls into town and everyone is getting sick… except for you. The consistent output of high voltage power from the logs on your fire makes you immune and illness bounces right off of you.

You have twice the amount of energy as most and don't have to take naps. Your hormones are balanced, your focus is crystal clear and you feel calm, energized and confident. You're also cranking out the work of five people, which gives you more time to vacation and pursue your dreams full time. Can you feel it?

As far-fetched as this may sound, if you open your eyes and ears and lock in the learnings of *The Power Diet* I can guarantee you'll see noticeable changes that are simply undeniable. Are you ready? Great, let's do it!

The 5 Power Food Categories

In order to boost your power to the max and help prevent mindless eating of imbalanced macros I've created six **"Power Food Categories."**

When crafting your next meal you can reference these or download *The Power Diet Master Guide* to meet your macros. I recommend adding from 3-5 of these Power Food Categories at each meal or snack. This includes the following:

Category 1 (a)	Power Veggies
Category 1 (b)	Prebiotic Veggies
Category 2	Nuts & Seeds
Category 3	Oils & Butter (Toppers)
Category 4	Starches & Sweets
Category 5	Protein

Choose foods from 3-5 Power Food Categories!

Below you'll find a break down of many of the power food choices from each category broken down into its respective macros including fat, net carbs (total carbs minus fiber) and protein.

Keep in mind; these examples represent the ideal macros for our hypothetical 160-pound individual with a 60-gram (2.1 ounces) requirement of protein per day. As such you'll need to make sure you modify these recommendations for your personal protein requirements.

If you're unsure what yours is make sure you revisit **"Calculate Your Optimal Protein Intake"** from earlier in this chapter.

Additionally, while we'll be splitting this daily total into two meals (30 grams of protein or 1.4 ounces per meal) you can split it into three meals or add a snack to reach your total requirement for daily macros.

Category 1(a) – Power Veggies (preferably organic)

Power veggies should be on your plate at most meals and can be eaten raw or cooked. Make sure you add least 1-3 sources from each of these and if you cook, lightly cook, steam, sauté or boil on low heat in order to retain power.

Add 1-3 "Power Veggies" to your meal!

Avocado

Fat	12
Net Carbs	1.3
Protein	1
Looks Like	½ medium size avocado

Broccoli

Fat	.2
Net Carbs	1.8
Protein	1.7
Looks Like	½ cup

Bok Choy

Fat	.1
Net Carbs	.4
Protein	1
Looks Like	½ cup steamed

Cauliflower

Fat	2
Net Carbs	.8
Protein	1.1
Looks Like	½ cup steamed

Collards

Fat	2
Net Carbs	1
Protein	1.7
Looks Like	½ cup steamed

Swiss Chard

Fat	1.6
Net Carbs	1.8
Protein	1.3
Looks Like	½ cup steamed

Kale

Fat	2
Net Carbs	2.3
Protein	1.3
Looks Like	½ cup steamed

Brussels Sprouts

Fat	2.2
Net Carbs	2.3
Protein	2
Looks Like	½ cup steamed

Carrots

Fat	.1
Net Carbs	2
Protein	.3
Looks Like	¼ cup chopped

Beetroot

Fat	1
Net Carbs	3.4
Protein	.7
Looks Like	¼ cup steamed

Sauerkraut or Kimchi

Fat	0
Net Carbs	1
Protein	0
Looks Like	1 tablespoon

Category 1(b) – Prebiotic Veggies (preferably organic)

While most vegetables have prebiotics that feed probiotics, I've opted to split category 1 into Part (a) and Part (b) to emphasize just how important it is to not only eat power veggies but to eat specific veggies which are highly concentrated with prebiotic power.

As such, category 1(b) represents some of the most potent and powerful prebiotic veggies available, which should be on your next plate.   With the exception of artichokes and asparagus, these should be eaten mostly raw and uncooked.

Add 1-3 "Prebiotic Veggies" to your meal!

Spirulina Smoothie Powder (organic, raw from BN Labs)

Fat	1
Net Carbs	1
Protein	4
Looks Like	1.5 teaspoons

Dandelion Greens

Fat	.2
Net Carbs	2
Protein	.7
Looks Like	½ cup raw chopped

Romaine, Butterleaf, Arugula and most other Lettuces

Fat	.14
Net Carbs	.5
Protein	.6
Looks Like	1 cup shredded

Artichoke

Fat	3
Net Carbs	4
Protein	4.2
Looks Like	1 medium steamed artichoke

Asparagus

Fat	2
Net Carbs	.3
Protein	2
Looks Like	½ cup steamed

Jicama

Fat	.03
Net Carbs	1.2
Protein	.3
Looks Like	¼ cup raw chopped

Radicchio

Fat	.03
Net Carbs	.4
Protein	.15
Looks Like	¼ cup shredded

Radishes

Fat	03
Net Carbs	.6
Protein	.2
Looks Like	¼ cup sliced

Category 2 – Nuts & Seeds (Preferably organic and raw)

Nuts can really boost your protein and fat intake and along with power veggies can provide smart alternatives to animal and fish sources. I recommend doing this one meal per day and see if you get an extra power boost.

Also, you can mix and match nuts and seeds depending on the meal you're making. For example, pine nuts taste great in Mediterranean dishes with oregano or olive oil while almonds and walnuts taste great in Asian cuisines with coconut oil.

Make sure you watch *The Power Diet* videos and learn how to make 10-minute power meals that feature favorite dishes like Indian, Japanese, Mexican, Italian and Thai!

Add 1-2 Nuts & Seeds to your meal!

Hemp Seeds

Fat	17
Net Carbs	0
Protein	14
Looks Like	1 handful or ¼ cup

Almonds (blanched)

Fat	18
Net Carbs	2
Protein	8
Looks Like	1 handful blanched or ¼ cup

Pistachio Nuts, Sesame Seeds

Fat	13
Net Carbs	3
Protein	6
Looks Like	1 handful, ¼ cup

Tahini

Fat	13
Net Carbs	5
Protein	6
Looks Like	2 tbsp.

Pine Nuts, Brazil Nuts, Hazelnuts

Fat	23
Net Carbs	1.6
Protein	5
Looks Like	1 handful or ¼ cup

Walnuts

Fat	16
Net Carbs	1
Protein	4
Looks Like	1 handful or ¼ cup

Almond Tortilla

Fat	5.5
Net Carbs	4
Protein	3
Looks Like	1 tortilla

Macadamia Nuts, Pecans

Fat	25
Net Carbs	2
Protein	2.5
Looks Like	1 handful or ¼ cup

Category 3 – Oils & Butter (Preferably organic and raw)

Oils are primarily fat and should be added to all meals. And while butter is technically a dairy product, in reality, its function as a "fat topper" is more similar to oil so we'll add it to this category.

As mentioned earlier, you'll be getting plenty of Omega-6 fats so it's important you make a conscious effort to get enough Omega-3 fats from grass fed butter and ghee, fish oil or krill oil supplements as well as walnut and hemp oil.

Add 1-2 Oils & Butter to your meal!

All Oils including Olive, Walnut, Coconut & MCT, Almond, Sesame, etc. (organic, extra virgin if possible)

Fat	14
Net Carbs	0
Protein	0
Looks Like	1 tablespoon

Butter (organic, grass fed, preferably raw)

Fat	11
Net Carbs	.1
Protein	.1
Looks Like	1 tablespoon

Category 4 – Starches & Sweets (preferably organic)

While starches are mostly carbs, they do contain some protein and can range anywhere from a fraction of a gram to 4 grams per serving.

Additionally, most of the starches in *The Power Diet* will also function as prebiotics; so if you can't get enough from your prebiotic veggies you can make up for it here.

Additionally, while some diets may create an entire category for fruit and sweets because they are primarily carbohydrates (stick fuel), we'll be limiting them and considering them in this category.

In order to get the maximum power boost, you'll want to add in 1-2 items from this category and if you need to cook just make sure you steam or use very low heat.

Warning Reminder

If you are overweight, have gut issues or are just starting out and have yet to become "fat adapted" (you burn sticks, not logs) you'll need to dial this one back since it's really easy to over consume carbs from starches and sweets.

Add 1-2 Starches to your meal!

Lentils

Fat	7
Net Carbs	12
Protein	8
Looks Like	½ cup pressure cooked

Adzuki Beans, Black Beans

Fat	.25
Net Carbs	10
Protein	10
Looks Like	¼ cup pressure cooked

Sweet Potato or Yam (organic steamed, boiled or baked)

Fat	.12
Net Carbs	7
Protein	1.1
Looks Like	¼ cup mashed

Shirataki Noodles

Fat	.01
Net Carbs	1.3
Protein	.2
Looks Like	½ cup

Cassava Tortilla

Fat	1.5
Net Carbs	12
Protein	1
Looks Like	1 tortilla

Cassava Taco Shells

Fat	7
Net Carbs	10
Protein	1
Looks Like	2 taco shells

Green Banana

Fat	0
Net Carbs	10
Protein	1
Looks Like	1 small green banana

Blueberries, Raspberries, Blackberries, Strawberries

Fat	0
Net Carbs	4.5
Protein	.3
Looks Like	¼ cup, a handful

Honey (organic, raw)

Fat	0
Net Carbs	6
Protein	0
Looks Like	1 teaspoon

Dark Chocolate (organic, 70% cacao)

Fat	3
Net Carbs	2
Protein	1
Looks Like	2 squares

Category 5 – Protein (Optional)

Animal and fish based food sources are mostly protein which can easily put you over the top and burry you in loads of pain. Make sure you familiarize yourself with how many grams you need and how many are in the power foods.

And again, in order to limit your consumption and boost your power I recommend cutting back by eating one animal based meal and one vegetarian based meal per day to start out.

Once you've done this for 30 days go back to animal and fish protein for all your meals for one week then all plant based for the following week and notice the difference. This will give you a really good idea of how your body responds with a power boost or power drain from these foods.

Add 1-2 animal or fish based sources to your meal!

Whey Smoothie Protein (grass fed from Dr. Mercola)

Fat	1
Net Carbs	7
Protein	10
Looks Like	1 scoop

Eggs

Fat	5
Net Carbs	.4
Protein	9
Looks Like	1 Large Egg

Sardines (Crown Prince Bristling in Water)

Fat	17
Net Carbs	0
Protein	14
Looks Like	3.5 ounces, 1 can in water, deck of cards

Sockeye Salmon (wild caught, low mercury)

Fat	5
Net Carbs	0
Protein	25
Looks Like	4 ounces, deck of cards

Tuna (wild caught, low mercury)

Fat	1
Net Carbs	0
Protein	18
Looks Like	3 ounces, canned, frozen or fresh, small deck of cards

Shrimp (wild caught, low mercury)

Fat	1
Net Carbs	.5
Protein	11
Looks Like	½ cup cooked

Cheese (organic, grass fed, preferably raw)

Fat	20
Net Carbs	3
Protein	18
Looks Like	3 ounces, 3 slices

Chicken

Fat	5
Net Carbs	0
Protein	16
Looks Like	3 ounces, small deck of cards

Beef, Lamb or Pork (organic grass fed)

Fat	15
Net Carbs	0
Protein	20
Looks Like	3 ounces, small deck of cards

Power Meal Scenarios

Now that you have a good idea of how to create a meal using the 5 Power Food Categories, let's revisit our scenario of that 160-pound individual and see what a typical two-meal day would look like on *The Power Diet*. Remember, you can swap out any of these options with other Power foods to meet your macros.

Meal 1 - Asian Power Bowl - Includes steamed broccoli and cauliflower rice topped with kimchi, tahini dressing and walnuts. Sweet potato with chocolate and butter on the side.

Category 1(a) – Power Veggies (organic)

Avocado

Fat	12
Net Carbs	1.3
Protein	1
Looks Like	½ medium size avocado

Broccoli

Fat	.2
Net Carbs	1.8
Protein	1.7
Looks Like	½ cup

Cauliflower

Fat	2
Net Carbs	.8
Protein	1.1
Looks Like	½ cup steamed

Kimchi

Fat	0
Net Carbs	1
Protein	0
Looks Like	1 tablespoon

Dandelion Greens

Fat	.2
Net Carbs	2
Protein	.7
Looks Like	½ cup raw chopped

Butterleaf Lettuce

Fat	.14
Net Carbs	.5
Protein	.6
Looks Like	1 cup shredded

Category 1(b) – Prebiotic Veggies (organic)

Jicama

Fat	.03
Net Carbs	1.2
Protein	.3
Looks Like	¼ cup raw chopped

Category 2 – Oils & Butter (Preferably organic and raw)

Olive Oil (organic, extra virgin if possible)

Fat	14
Net Carbs	0
Protein	0
Looks Like	1 tablespoon

Butter (organic, grass fed, preferably raw)

Fat	5
Net Carbs	0
Protein	0
Looks Like	1 teaspoon

Category 3 – Nuts & Seeds (Preferably organic and raw)

Tahini

Fat	13
Net Carbs	5
Protein	6
Looks Like	2 tbsp.

Walnuts

Fat	16
Net Carbs	1
Protein	4
Looks Like	1 handful or ¼ cup

Dark Chocolate (organic, 70% cacao)

Fat	3
Net Carbs	2
Protein	1
Looks Like	2 squares

Sweet Potato (organic steamed, boiled or baked)

Fat	.12
Net Carbs	7
Protein	1.1
Looks Like	¼ cup mashed

Sockeye Salmon (wild caught, low mercury)

Fat	5
Net Carbs	0
Protein	25
Looks Like	4 ounces, small deck of cards

Total Macros

Now let's take a look at the total for each macro and see if it's in our target range.

Fat	116 (58 x 2 = 116)
Net Carbs	24
Protein	37
Tastes Like	Heaven!

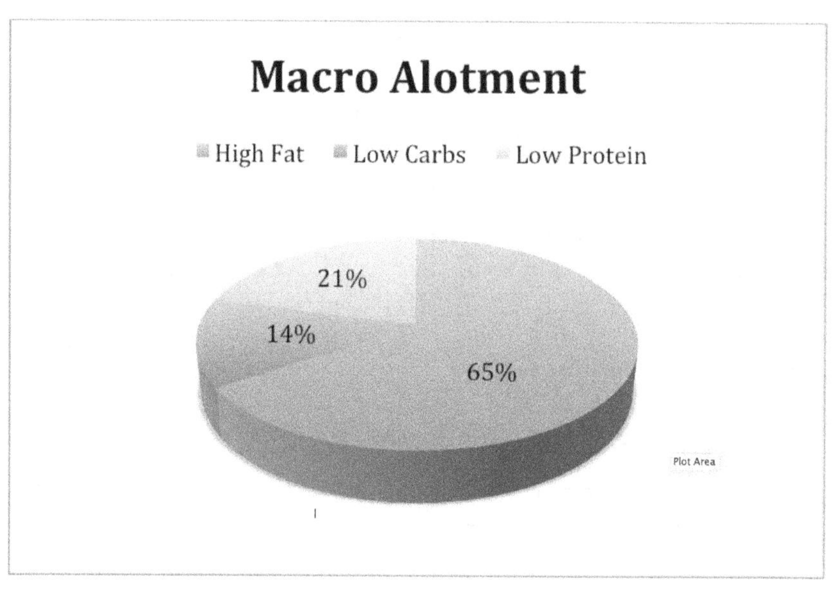

As you can see this meal has met the macro requirements for *The Power Diet*. And remember, since fat has twice the calories of both protein and carbs I doubled the total fat in order to arrive at the true macro percentage.
As you can imagine this meal is deliciously decadent but incredibly nutritious and satisfying. After you eat this you won't have any cravings.   And if you're thinking it takes a lot of time, forget it! This and many other power meals can be found in *The Power Diet* "10 Minute Meal" video library, which I highly recommend you check out at:
https://chadscottcoaching.com/power-diet
   Now let's move on to our next meal of the day. I think you're really gonna love this one.

Meal 2 - Mexican Fiesta Tacos - with cauliflower rice, pine nuts, adzuki beans, avocado, chard and jicama in cassava taco shells

Category 1(a) – Power Veggies (organic)

Avocado

Fat	12
Net Carbs	1.3
Protein	1
Looks Like	½ medium size avocado

Cauliflower

Fat	2
Net Carbs	.8
Protein	1.1
Looks Like	½ cup steamed

Swiss Chard

Fat	1.6
Net Carbs	1.8
Protein	1.3
Looks Like	½ cup

Category 1(b) – Prebiotic Veggies (organic)

Romaine Lettuce

Fat	.14
Net Carbs	1.5
Protein	.6
Looks Like	1 cup shredded

Jicama

Fat	0
Net Carbs	1.3
Protein	.3
Looks Like	¼ cup chopped

Category 2 – Oils & Butter (Preferably organic and raw)

Olive Oil (organic, extra virgin if possible)

Fat	14
Net Carbs	0
Protein	0
Looks Like	1 tablespoon

Dark Chocolate (organic, 70% cacao)

Fat	3
Net Carbs	2
Protein	1
Looks Like	2 squares

Category 3 – Nuts & Seeds (Preferably organic and raw)

Pine Nuts

Fat	23
Net Carbs	1.6
Protein	5
Looks Like	1 handful or ¼ cup

Category 4 – Starches (organic)

Adzuki Beans or Black Beans

Fat	.25
Net Carbs	10
Protein	10
Looks Like	¼ cup pressure cooked

Cassava Taco Shells

Fat	7
Net Carbs	11
Protein	1
Looks Like	2 taco shells

Total Macros

Fat	124 (62 x 2 = 124)
Net Carbs	31
Protein	21
Tastes Like	A Fiesta in your mouth!

Now let's take a look at the total for each macro and see if it's in our target range.

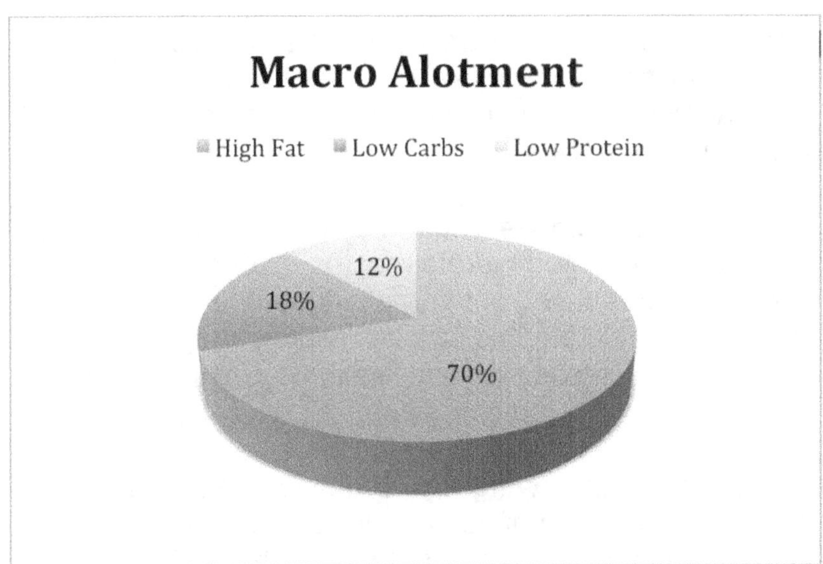

As you can see this meal is high in fat and low in both carbs and protein - within our target range for the day.

And while you can make meals that do not fall within *The Power Diet* macro ranges, this isn't a license to be extreme as this will most likely throw a bomb in your belly and send you to the couch or worse the hospital. What's most important here is stay make sure you never fall out of the target range by more than 3-5 percent.

Follow The Power Diet Protocol

If you simply follow *The Power Diet* protocol by adding foods from 3-5 of the power food categories at each meal and you experiment by adding and subtracting from your macros, you will find your sweet spot and not only achieve maximum power throughout the day but you kill off the cravings, bulletproof your immune system and feel completely satisfied from eating delicious meals.

Take Action – Hit Your Quantity Target

Now that you're more familiar with the macro foods for maximum power let's recap so you don't forget.
    If you are just starting off you'll need to first determine if you are at your ideal weight.

- If you need to **lose weight**, make sure you shoot for the lower range of carbohydrate macros (about 10% of total macros) and reduce your carbohydrate intake by 10-20%. To accelerate this process make sure you invest in an optimized fitness program like *Fired Up* and follow the cutting phase recommendations.

- If you need to **gain weight or bulk**, you'll need to shoot for the higher range of carbohydrate macros (up to 30%) and increase your carbohydrate intake by 10-20%. To accelerate this process use the *Fired Up* program and follow the bulking phase recommendations.

- If you are at your **ideal weight** follow *The Power Diet and Fired Up* protocols as follows:

✓   High Fat - 50-70% of calories from healthy fats
✓   Low Carbs - 10-30% of calories from carbs.
✓   Low Protein - 10-20% of calories from protein

Other Tools To Decipher Macros

As you can see, there is quite a bit of crossover between the three macros. So if you're relatively new to nutrition science and eyeballing food to determine its percentage of carbs vs. fats vs. protein is challenging, I highly recommend using a couple of the following resources:

The Power Diet Video Library – The Power Diet video library shows you step-by-step how to cook 10 minute mouth watering meals that will make you feel fully nourished and alive with power. Once you learn these basic recipes you can use them for the rest of your life without having to think about measurements or calculations. Also, if you dine out frequently, these will help when it comes time to order. Check it out here: www.ChadScottCoaching.com/power-diet

My Fitness Pal – This website allows you to input foods and brands and get a readout of macros. Review it here: https://www.myfitnesspal.com/

Fat Secret – This free website allows you to check the grams of carbs, fats and protein in most foods. Check it out here: https://www.fatsecret.com/calories-nutrition

Focus On Quality 1st and Quantity 2nd

Don't worry about getting your macros exact; instead, focus on the quality of your food until you're feeling you can eat mostly power boosting foods. Once you're feeling a boost start experiment with quantity until you find your sweet spot.

Ditch Mindless Eating

Assuming you have not overeaten, the next thing you'll need to do is experiment with different quantities in order to find your sweet spot of optimum power and sustained energy.

Most importantly, it's time to ditch the mindless eating by simply slapping whatever you have available on your plate. Instead, mindfully manage your macros and listen to your mind and body. Assuming you're eating mostly power boosting foods and you're well rested if you have digestion issues or feel off in available energy or concentration levels you can simply add or subtract from your macros to find your sweet spot of optimum power and energy! And remember your new mantra:

Each time I eat, I am mindful of my macros!

Pillar 3 - Frequency

Alas, we've come to the third and final pillar of the power diet. Frequency is, quite simply, how often you eat, which more often than not, leads to "Overkill" or more appropriately "Overeating" and "Overweight."

Confusingly, when it comes to frequency, there is no shortage of recommendations in the diet world, many of which have led to the devastating effects of inflammation, obesity and a host of other life crushing diseases.

For example, for decades many nutritionists have been recommending three meals and two snacks a day to consistently supply calories and stave off any feelings of hunger. Unfortunately, as Hippocrates once warned:

"Everything in excess is opposed to nature"

Interestingly enough, what was deemed as excess thousands of years ago holds true even more so today. Studies confirm overconsumption of food as a primary contributor to an obesity epidemic, which (as of this writing) represents roughly 40% of the United States' population of adults over 20 years old.[153]

This should be a wake up call to take action and lose weight, especially considering the fact that, as you learned earlier, roughly one out of every two hospitalizations for the Coronavirus worldwide pandemic were people who were overweight or obese.

And while you may have been conditioned to believe that breakfast is the most important meal of the day, to be eaten shortly after you wake up, you may be surprised to find out this is based more on myth than science. And let's not forget about all those amazing benefits that occur when you are not constantly taxing your body with the digestion and assimilation of foods.

If you simply think about the process of eating or do a little research on the subject, you'll find that the process of breaking down, digesting, and assimilating food uses a lot of energy,[154] which brings us back to that big question about your last meal:

Did This Food Give Me Power Or Take It Away?

If you eat and you feel drained of power, if you are overweight, if you get sick frequently, if you have cravings, feel irritable or anxious there's a really good chance you are eating too frequently.

Regrettably, when you eat too frequently, you're body has to work overtime, which taxes every system in your body and mind. So on top of the normal functions like respiration, circulation and detoxification, when you eat too frequently your body has to constantly digest and assimilate food, which makes your immune system less effective. And according to the American Academy of Neurology, this overtime work costs you in brain impairment.[155]

Yes, unfortunately, one of the first things to go is your brain and its ability to think, which could then lead to dementia or even Alzheimer's.

But that's just the beginning, as eating too frequently also leads to obesity, cancer, heart disease and a host of other illnesses.[156]

So what's the solution?

Intermittent Fasting (IF)

Over the last 20 years of my life I've been obsessed with a relentless pursuit of the ultimate diet for optimum performance and taste. During this time I've studied all the major breakthroughs in nutritional science and experimented with power packed super foods and cutting edge supplements. And while much of what I learned has made a profound impact on my overall health, nothing has helped me restore and create more power than by doing one seemingly crazy thing – eat less frequently!

Interestingly, this one thing also happens to be the most simple and affordable solution ever discovered in the history of health.

Yes, eating less frequently, otherwise known as fasting, is an absolute game changer. For example, I used to experience long bouts battling a painful and bloated gut even after I removed toxic lectins from my diet. To remedy the situation I would take high-powered probiotics, prebiotics, eat a streamlined diet and ditch all the sugar but nothing seemed to completely eliminate the problem.

Since I experienced so much pain for so many years when I found out about the power of fasting, naturally I was curious and game to try it. And boy did it work.

By simply not eating any food for 24 hours I was able to "reset my microbiome" and regrow my forest of life giving microbes.

Many health experts, already mentioned in this book, like Dr. Gundry, Dr. Mercola, Mark Sisson and Dave Asprey also recommend this as a powerful health strategy to use for optimizing performance and enhancing immunity and there's a really good reason.

Effectively, when your microbiome is unimpeded by constant digestion and assimilation of food, this frees up an army of soldiers who can then take control and virtually wipe out any unwanted invaders.

For me, fasting was like a miracle! Each time I used this strategy I was able to completely wipe out any harmful bacteria, free myself of stomach pain and boost my health to a whole new level.

At this point, I can just hear the rumblings of readers thinking about how painful it would be to stop eating for a whole 24 hours. But before you freak out and put the book down, first just take a deep breath and remember to stay open to everything and attached to nothing.

Second, you should know by now that you're not going to die if you don't eat right away. In fact, Mahatma Gandhi survived 21 days with zero food (and low body fat) and studies cite several hunger strikes that lasted 21-40 days with zero food.[157]

And third, you should know that a 24-48 hour fast is a longer fast, which I only do a few times a year. For the most part, we'll be using a much more simple and sustainable strategy in *The Power Diet*.

It's also important to recognize that millions of people practice fasting as a religious tradition and look forward to its benefits several times a year.

Perhaps even more revealing is how fasting has been used by the medical community as a health strategy to heal ailments ranging from arthritis to heart disease to leaky gut and everything in between.

Additional studies back this up and have shown that fasting has the power to:

- Decrease blood pressure, triglycerides, total cholesterol and LDL cholesterol.[158]
- Reduce risk of neurodegenerative disorders like Alzheimer's and Parkinson's.[159] [160]
- Decrease levels of inflammatory markers and autoimmune disorders like arthritis.[161]
- Decrease instances of diabetes by lowering blood sugar and insulin.[162]

And the list goes on. Essentially, in order to give your body the time it needs to recover and rebuild more strength, muscle, memory, agility, clarity, sexual potency and overall power you'll need to stop eating for longer periods of time.

Naturally, this relates back to metabolic flexibility and ketosis, which we'll be using in *The Power Diet* to give your mind and body ample time to recover and rebuild to maximum power.

To do this, we'll be using one of the most powerful eating strategies ever created – Intermittent Fasting.

Intermittent fasting allows you to burn enough fat to use for energy while releasing a level of toxins that your body can handle. And according to Dr. Joe Mercola, best selling author of *Fat For Fuel*:

"Combining intermittent fasting with cyclical ketosis is one of the fastest ways to increase metabolic flexibility. It gets your body used to using the fuel that's available, and your system won't go into a panic whenever one or the other fuel type (glucose or fat) isn't available."

According to studies, it takes roughly 12 hours to turn ketosis on but you'll need a good 2 hours in this fat burning mode to start getting the benefits.[163] In this state, your body starts to break down and burn fat as its primary fuel source. So in *The Power Diet,* you'll be fasting between 12 and 18 hours per day and eating during a 6-10 hour window for men and an 8-12 hour window for women.

IF for Women Vs. Men

We talked earlier about women's unique reproductive needs which can make them highly sensitive to calorie restriction but it's important to understand that when it comes to fasting, this is even more important.

Specifically, when calorie consumption is low from fasting for too long or too frequently, a small part of your brain called the hypothalamus is affected. This can, in turn, disrupt the secretion of gonadotropin-releasing hormone (GnRH), a hormone that helps release two female reproductive hormones: luteinizing hormone (LH) and follicle stimulating hormone (FSH).[164] [165]

Unfortunately, when these two hormones cannot communicate with the ovaries, women run the risk of irregular periods, infertility, poor bone health and other not so fun stuff.[166]

Because of this extra sensitivity to calorie restriction, I recommend women stay within an eating window of 8-12 hours, while men can close that window further to 6-10 hours of eating time per day.

Warning: If you're pregnant or nursing I recommend NOT fasting more than 12 hours. Your kid needs food so please, feed them adequately!

And for those that are not pregnant or nursing, if you're at all worried about not eating as frequently just remember, an increase in fasting time allows your body time to restore its natural balance and kick on several healing mechanisms you simply can't get when you eat too frequently.

Intermittent Fasting Boosters

Since IF is so critical to boosting your power, let's talk more about some of the life lifting benefits. But again, in order to make this a lifetime habit, don't just read them; instead, imagine yourself living with them.

Save Your Hard Earned Dollars

This might be obvious but it's a great side effect of intermittent fasting. Just imagine not having to go to the store and buy snacks all the time or not having to pay for breakfast every day because your newly increased fat intake from The Power Diet allows you to burn clean logs all the way up to lunch. You'll end up saving a lot of money.

Save Precious Time

Can you imagine not having to spend so much time driving to restaurants, waiting for food or spend hours on end preparing them yourself and the time you'll free up time to work on your passions?

And to assist you in cutting down your meal prep time, *The Power Diet* contains a <u>video library</u> of "10 minute meals" that will show you step-by-step how to make mouthwatering meals in just minutes.

Enjoy Food Even More with Gratitude

Just because you save time, money and stress less about food doesn't mean you'll enjoy it less. In fact, most people who've made the switch to *The Power Diet* enjoy food more.

To put this into perspective, imagine a drug addict or in this case a Carboholic (someone addicted to carbohydrates). When you continue ingesting something repetitively, eventually, you become desensitized to its effects. In economics, this is called "The Law of Diminishing Returns."

Similarly, when you eat too frequently you become desensitized, not only to the taste of food but also the feelings of gratitude.[167]

Fortunately, when you moderate consumption with intermittent fasting you have a greater appreciation for tastes and overall abundance in life.

To boost your gratitude power and enjoy food even more, I recommend that before you eat every meal you give thanks to everything and everyone that took part in bringing the food to your plate. If you can get in the habit of giving thanks for your food you'll more than likely eat more slowly and enjoy it more!

Now imagine a delicious plate of food in front of you as you place your hands over it to feel its power. Then imagine smelling all the sweet and savory smells while repeating the following prayer of gratitude:

"Thank you for the sunshine, the soil, the farmers and everyone who took part in bringing this food to my plate, may it nourish and heal me."

Reverse Your Age & Increase Power With Autophagy

In 2016 Nobel Laureate Yoshinori Ohsumi discovered and elucidated mechanisms underlying autophagy, a fundamental process for degrading and recycling cellular components.

If you're not already familiar with this word "autophagy" it originates from the Greek words auto, meaning "self", and phagein, meaning, "to eat". Thus, autophagy denotes "self eating," which is highly significant since studies show:

"Autophagy allows cell waste and damaged material in the cell to be recycled into energy or new proteins. ... If cancer cells want to multiply, they use autophagy to burn up waste material for energy to grow." [168]

In other words, autophagy burns up waste material before cancer cells can use it to multiply. And while the science is still new here, studies show the process of autophagy holds great promise for cancer treatment.[169]

While autophagy could be one of the greatest discoveries of modern day medicine (or more accurately - no medicine) there's a catch to acquiring it. Turns out, autophagy is most effective during fasting and overeating protein or carbs turns it off.[170] Did you catch that? This is so important I'll repeat it:

Autophagy is most effective during fasting and overeating protein or carbs turns it off!

So how long do you need to fast to turn on autophagy?

While the science differs from source to source, according to Dr. Joseph Mercola you need to fast for roughly 18 hours to start seeing the benefits of autophagy, while others claim it takes a minimum of 24 hours.[171]

While it's clear autophagy becomes more pronounced deeper into a fast, since this has yet to become an exact science, the more important thing to focus on here is consistency over time. If you can stick to a 6-10 hour window consistently, over time you'll see massive benefits from this power player.

Additionally, once you become fat adapted, you can fast for 24-48 hours a few times per year to really take advantage of autophagy and enjoy growth hormone levels as much as five times as high as when you started your fast.[172] So for 24-48 hours, the only thing you'll be ingesting would be water, tea or coffee, which doesn't have protein or carbs.

Personally, I do 3-6 longer fasts between 24 and 48 hours each year and I highly recommend you do this as well, especially if you suffer from any autoimmune disorders like arthritis, psoriasis or gut issues like leaky gut.

You can simply start with a 24 hour fast, which will be a breeze once you become fat adapted.

Lastly, as an added bonus, when you invest in a fitness program like Fired Up, according to animal studies exercise may also play a significant role in further inducing autophagy.[173]

Less Stress

It's a well-known fact that too much stress can be worse for your health than smoking, eating junk food and a sedentary lifestyle combined. Fortunately, when you know (scientifically and experiential) that you're not going to die from fasting for short periods of time and don't have to think about where you're next meal or snack is coming from, you let go of all the stress associated with scarcity and needing to eat all the time.

Now can you imagine a time where you were stressed out because you forgot to bring lunch or you missed lunch or you couldn't find a good meal?

Now go ahead and re-imagine that same scenario but instead of panicking; this time you knew with 100% certainty that you weren't going to die, in fact, you looked forward to skipping that meal because the absence of food allowed you go into a state of autophagy and clean out some dead toxic debris accumulated from the weekend, which was killing your power.

Smooth Transition From Stick Burner To Log Burner

Most nutrition experts find that it takes between 30-60 days
to gain metabolic flexibility with intermittent fasting. And
while I'll be guiding you step-by-step, to make this transition
as smooth as possible, it's crucial you understand that you
may experience a few bumps along the road.

During this period, people who don't know what they're
doing experience overwhelming cravings for carbs,
increased irritability, headaches and what's widely known as
"The Keto Flu."

Additional signs to be aware of are itchy red dots or
splotchy red patches on various parts of your body
(underarms and crotch are common). If this happens to you
don't worry; this is your body's natural process of getting rid
of all those toxins, which are draining your power.

The good news is, I'm going to give you the secret power
strategies for avoiding most of these unpleasant side effects,
so once you come out of this detoxification phase, you'll start
feeling superpowers, devoid of cravings, and loaded with
energy, brainpower, and an elevated mood.

Your Eating Window

Your eating window is the amount of time during a 24-hour
period you can eat. *The Power Diet* program provides a
broad eating window of 6-10 hours for men and 8-12 hours
for women, which can be modified depending on various
circumstances.

What Is The Ideal Eating Window For Me?

The degree you raise or lower this window will depend on
the following:

Are You Male or Female - If you are a male you can
experiment with a wide range from 6-10 hours of eating time
and if you're a woman you'll want to open that up a couple of
hours and experiment within an 8-12 hour range.

What's Your Body Type –Do you gain weight easily? If you tend to gain weight fast, consider shortening your eating window by doing the recommended 8-week drawdown (explained shortly) until you get to a 6-8 hour window for men or an 8-10 hour window for women.

What Are Your Goals – Is your goal to maximize power and reverse the aging process with more autophagy? For example, if you do not struggle with weight gain but your goal is to experience all the benefits from ketosis and autophagy explained earlier, you will also need to complete the recommended 8-week drawdown until you reach a 6-10 hour window for men or an 8-12 hour window for women.

Cycle Off 1-2 Days – If you choose to cycle off of High Fat and Low Carb, Low Protein for one or two days per week by increasing carb and protein consumption you can open your eating window up to 12 hours regardless of sex.

How Do You Feel – How does your eating window make you feel long-term (over a 60-day period)? Once you become a fat adapted log burner and you feel really good with a window that falls somewhere in *The Power Diet* recommended ranges (6-10 hours for men or 8-12 for women), you can stick with this and get most of the benefits from *The Power Diet*. But again, I encourage you to explore within the recommended ranges and continue to seek out your personal sweet spot that works best for your personal circumstances.

Longer Fasts – I mentioned how I solved what I considered an unsolvable health issue with a longer 24-48 hour fast. And once you become a fat adapted log burner you too can employ this strategy when you feel like nothing is working to solve a gut issue or autoimmune disorder.
Keep in mind, I'm not a doctor and I make no claim as to the efficacy of fasting from a medical standpoint. But I can say with 100% certainty that from my personal experience, a 24-48 hour fast can work miracles in boosting your health so I advise all my clients to do this at least 2-4 times per year.

In addition, I also do a 24-48 hour fast once or twice a year and once you are fully fat adapted you can try this as well. Just make sure if you do a longer fast you do not go past 3 days, as this seems to be the point where benefits go down and damage goes up.

And while you'll want to make sure you drink plenty of water during your fast, you can also add small amounts of lemon, lime, salt and trace minerals to your water to ease the burden of brain fog and lift your pH level.

Lastly, while it's optional and may slightly reduce some of the benefits of fasting, you can add some ketone fat toppers to your tea and coffee such as MCT Oil, coconut oil or grass fed butter. See our resources page for more recommendations.

The 8-Week Drawdown

If your body is not used to burning ketones and you are not yet metabolically flexible (fat adapted), you'll need to draw down your eating window over time. If on the other hand, you simply rush into ketosis with the desire to lose as many pounds as quickly as possible, you could experience some unpleasant side effects like nausea, headaches and insomnia.

To answer this challenge I've created an 8-week program that allows you to gradually decrease (draw down) your eating window while avoiding most of the unpleasant side effects.

While not everyone will arrive at the same drawdown window, **I do recommend everyone start with a gradual drawdown** in order to ease into ketosis. Accordingly, make sure you take action on the following drawdown program.

Week 1-2 Eliminate Power Drains
Eating Window: Men 9-10 Hrs. Women 10-12 Hrs.
Days Per Week: 5-7

During weeks 1-2 you'll first need to begin eliminating the power draining foods and toxins and stick to the power boost and power limit foods. Make sure you download *The Power Diet Master Guide* and put it on your refrigerator as well as on your smartphone for quick access.

Download: https://chadscottcoaching.com/PD-Master-G.jpg

During these first two weeks, you can eat during a flexible window (9-10 hours for men and 10-12 for women). Let's take a look at what a hypothetical day would look like.

Wake up at 7:00 am and drink water, tea or coffee then slurp down a super green fat smoothie at 9:00 or 10:00 am followed by lunch at 12:00 or 1:00 pm. You could potentially have a small high fat snack around 3:00 pm if you are truly hungry, which would then be followed by dinner as your last meal around 6:00 or 7:00 pm.

Just keep in mind, if you wake up at 5:00 am you can experiment by moving this timetable up a couple of hours.

Once you finish these first two weeks, if you feel your energy levels are good and you do not have major cleansing reactions, continue on to the next drawdown, otherwise stay here and use the action strategies at the end of this chapter until symptoms clear up.

Week 3-4 Limit The Power Limits
Eating Window: Men 8-9 Hrs. Women 9-11 Hrs.
Days Per Week: 5-7

In your third and fourth week, you'll have eliminated most if not all of the power drains, which means it's now time to start limiting the "Power Limit" foods to 1-3 days per week.

During these next couple weeks, you'll close your eating window another hour and continue transitioning from stick burner to log burner, which may require some additional hacks to avoid cravings and brain fog. We'll cover those in our action steps shortly. For now, just know this will extend your morning fast, so let's take a look at what a typical day would look like.

Wake up and drink water, tea or coffee for a few hours (possibly with a fat topper), then drink a power smoothie at 10:00 or 11:00 am followed by lunch at 1:00 or 2:00 pm.

You could have a small high fat snack if you are truly hungry at around 3:00 pm, which would be followed by dinner as your last meal around 6:00 or 7:00 pm.

If you feel your energy levels are good and you do not have major cleansing reactions, continue on to the next drawdown, otherwise stay here and use the recommended "Pain Free Transition Strategies" coming up shortly until symptoms clear up.

Week 5-6 Focus On The Power Boosts
Eating Window: M 7-8 Hrs. W 8-10 Hrs.
Days Per Week: 5-7

In your second month on *The Power Diet,* you'll have eliminated all the power drains, limited the power limits and begun focusing primarily on power boosting foods.

For these next two weeks, you'll need to draw down your eating window by another hour (M 7-8 Hrs. W 8-10 Hrs.) but since you're burning bigger and bigger branches (soon to be logs) things should start getting a little easier here. Let's take a look at an example of a typical day.

Wake up, drink some water, tea or coffee (possibly with a fat topper) skip breakfast and eat lunch at 11:00 am or 12:00 pm. This could potentially be followed by a small high fat snack at 3:00 pm with dinner as your last meal at 6:00 or 7:00 pm.

If you feel your energy levels are good and you do not have major cleansing reactions, continue on to the next drawdown, otherwise stay here and make sure you follow the "Pain Free Transition Strategies" coming up shortly.

Week 7-8 The Lifetime Habit Begins
Eating Window: M 6-7 Hrs. W 8-9 Hrs.
Days Per Week: 5-7

If you've followed *The Power Diet* protocol for the last six weeks it's time to get excited, because your last two weeks should be on cruise control.

Yes, you have one final optional drawdown of one hour but since you're burning decent size logs this shouldn't be much of a challenge.

And if cruise control sounds cool, just imagine being on cruise control for the rest of your life. Yes, it is possible but only if you can get to the 60-day mark or beyond as studies show it takes an average of 66 days to form a new habit.[174]

Thankfully, once you form a habit of eating the right quality, quantity and frequency recommended in *The Power Diet* you won't want to turn back because you'll start feeling the powerful effects of autophagy, age reversal, superhuman healing powers, laser-like focus and increased libido! Why would anyone want to turn their back on that?

So what does this final two weeks look like?

You'll wake up and drink some water, tea or coffee, perhaps with a fat topper and skip breakfast. Then around 12:00 or 1:00 pm you'll eat lunch with a potential snack around 3:00 pm followed by dinner as your last meal around 7:00 pm – easy peasy!

Special Warning: Women who are still fertile should take extra precaution not to close your eating window beyond 8 hours.

What To Do After The 8-Week Drawdown

If you eventually make it here (6-8 hour window for men 8-9 for women) you can stay as long as you like.

Congrats and welcome to the log burning club!

Regardless of how far you draw down your eating window, I encourage you to experiment with the recommended ranges (6-10 hours for men and 8-12 for women) and be objective about what really feels good for you long-term.

For example, if you never made it to the 6-8 hour window and never really experienced autophagy how can you ever really be objective and say it did not work for you?

In contrast, if you did make it to the 6-8 hour window for a good 30 days and followed all the action items but did not receive any worthwhile benefits, perhaps you need to be more flexible and try a different window that works better for your circumstances.

The key here is to be objective and experiment long-term with different options within the recommended ranges to truly see what really boosts or drains your power. So in addition to experimenting with your eating window, I highly encourage you to experiment with your macros by adding and subtracting fat, carbs and protein within the recommended ranges to find your ultimate sweet spot of happy eating and maximum power.

And remember, this is a flexible program, so if for some reason you fall off the wagon for a week or two, you can always jump back on without losing too much of your progress.

Don't Flood The Tank!

Clearly, there are massive benefits to limiting the frequency of food consumption as a daily strategy but you can boost your power and immunity even further by limiting the amount of food consumed at each individual meal.

Similar to a car, when you flood the tank most processes and operations that keep you alive start to shut down and once again you're on the sidelines relegated to the couch.

Question: How do you eat?

If you're confused about this question or thinking along the lines of: "I pick it up and I eat it," this could be another great opportunity to increase your power.

Essentially, this brings us back to our "Mindful Eating" strategy and allows you to not only taste food and enjoy it but more importantly to digest it and take advantage of its power producing nutrients (AKA assimilation). Let's take a look at some of the most important mindful eating strategies with some action.

Take Action

To imprint this lesson into your brain and really apply it to your life, go ahead and transport yourself to the last holiday or birthday party where you clearly ate too much. Got one in mind?

Can you remember how you felt? Can you remember what took you over the top?

Perhaps the 32 ounce steak, the apple pie, the cookies, the extra helping of potatoes or maybe it was just that TV show you got lost in and mindlessly ate your way to the bottom of a bucket of ice cream.

And what was your mobility like? How about your mind? Were you able to think clearly and work on your passions? Did you feel like singing and dancing or slamming a coffee and melting into a couch?

Whatever you felt, it's important to understand that the same problems and diseases that occur from eating too frequently also apply to eating too much at one meal.

Stop Eating At 90% Capacity

To remedy this challenge you'll need to stop eating when you hit 90% of the maximum capacity of what your stomach can hold. So right now let's pause and return to that time you overloaded your gut with too much food.

Do you remember a voice in the back of your head asking you something like: "should I eat more," "maybe I should stop eating," or "do I really need more food?"

Whether you remember or not, from here on out you'll need to make a commitment to honor that voice; it means STOP! This is your intuition telling you to stop eating so you don't flood the tank and become a bloated bench warmer tied to a TV clicker and a couch. So remember:

Stop eating when you are 90% full!

Eat Small Desserts or Wait To Eat Dessert

More often than not, I find a great majority of people who struggle with overeating are addicted to sweets or more appropriately, the hit of serotonin that accompanies it. Since banning all sweets is simply unsustainable long-term, I recommend doing one of two things.

1) Stop eating at 80-90% of capacity and give yourself a healthy treat like a couple squares of raw chocolate or any other recommended desserts from our <u>resources section</u>. By purchasing the right power desserts you'll be able to satisfy your sweet tooth and bypass the surge of insulin and it's accompanying power drain.

2) Stop eating at 90% of capacity and wait about an hour to assess whether or not you really need any more food. This is really important since digestion takes time and it's difficult to know whether or not you've eaten enough to be satiated.

And keep in mind the good news here. If you hold off on eating more food and an hour or two later begin to feel true hunger arise, you can eat anytime within your window. So remember this:

Eat small desserts or wait to eat dessert!

If You Are Sick Stop At 80% Capacity!

Have you ever been sick with a cold or the flu and noticed your symptoms worsen when you ate sugar or carbs or just too much food in general?

When you're sick, your body is working overtime sending white blood cell soldiers and immune bombs to fight off the invaders, which means it doesn't have much power left to digest and assimilate food, especially refined sugars. In fact, according to studies, when you feed yourself too much sugar your white blood cells lose power and can't fight off the invaders.[175]

If you ever find yourself in this position, make sure you eliminate sugary foods and stick to *The Power Diet* recommendations. Additionally, you'll need to dial down your overall consumption of food to a couple meals a day and make sure you stop eating when you are 80% full.   This means you should be slightly hungry when you finish your meal.

This is important, as it will allow your digestive system to redirect minimal resources towards assimilation and maximal resources toward winning the battle against any potential illness. So remember:

If you are sick stop eating when you are 80% full!

Eat Slowly And Mindfully

If you grew up with a lot of siblings or regularly dine at a table full of people who look like raving dogs with forks and knives you may suffer from FOMO (fear of missing out), which may have conditioned you to believe you would starve to death if you didn't eat fast enough and get your share.

Yes, eating too fast has a huge effect on your power or lack thereof, and according to studies leaves you at a significantly higher risk of becoming obese, getting diabetes and/or heart disease than if you simply slowed down.[176]

And if being overweight and more susceptible to illness doesn't motivate you to slow down perhaps knowing that all that food you just ate could erupt in a fiery explosion from your gut shortly after you consumed it will. According to multiple studies, eating too fast can lead to GERD or acid reflux, a not so fun reaction to rapid shoveling of food down your throat.[177]

Simply not flooding the tank and stopping after you become 80-90% full will definitely help with this challenge but you'll need to slow down if you are to actually digest, assimilate and gain real power from the food you consume.

To do this I recommend finding your ideal bite with all the ingredients you want in your mouth for maximum flavor, then chew that bite until it's liquid and don't bother to take another bite until you finish the one that's in your mouth.

Of course, slowing down your eating plays directly into not flooding the tank due to the fact that when you eat slowly the signals of ghrelin and leptin (hungry and full) have time to synch up and give you a much more accurate reading. Ultimately, when these signals are synched up you'll have a much easier time identifying that 80-90% level and be able to stop eating before you flood the tank.

Last but certainly not least, eating slowly allows you to magnify that "gratitude" benefit we talked about in intermittent fasting.

By turning off your TV, sitting down and turning on some music, instead of activating your fight or flight mechanism which creates more stress and makes digestion even more difficult, according to studies, you'll activate your parasympathetic nervous system, which is responsible for rest and digest.[178]

And as a reminder, this is a perfect time to practice gratitude by contemplating and acknowledging how long it took to grow your food, all the farmers that tended to the garden or fed the animals, and the people that prepared it and brought it to your table.

This may sound simple, but it's highly effective and without a doubt a strategy you should employ every time you sit down to eat. So remember:

Eat slowly and mindfully!

Summary of Recommendations

Now that you understand the 8-week drawdown and how to eat when you actually sit down for your next meal let's go ahead and summarize what we know so far about eating frequency.

5-7 Day Cycle

Choose any 5-7 days per week to eat predominantly healthy fats while reducing carbs and protein. Try to stay in the following macro ranges:

✓ High Fat - 50-70 %
✓ Med Carbs - 10-30 %
✓ Low Protein - 10-20 %
✓ Eating Window - Men 6-10 hours / Women 8-12
✓ Eat Slow and Stop Eating when you reach 80-90% of capacity

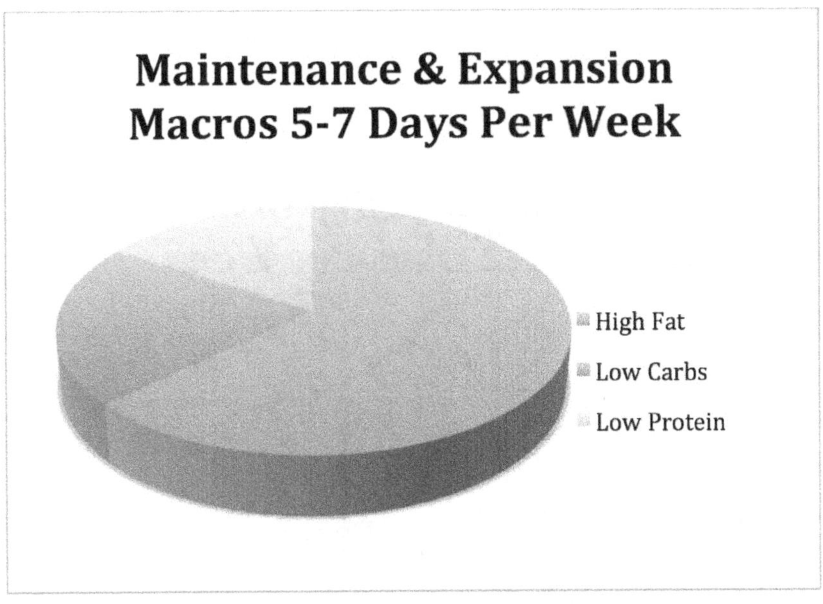

1-2 Day Cycle Off (Optional)

You can optionally cycle off high fat by lowering fat and increasing both carbs and protein 1-2 days per week to provide more flexible eating.

If you do this just make sure you aren't binging on carbs and protein but rather slightly boosting your intake 1-2 days a week. The following would be a realistic shift in your macros on those days.

✓ Med Fat - 30-50 % of calories from healthy fats
✓ Med Carb - 20-40 % of calories from carbs
✓ Low Protein - 20-30 % of calories from protein
✓ Eating Window - 8-12 hours (men and women)
✓ Eat Slow and Stop Eating when you reach 80-90% of capacity

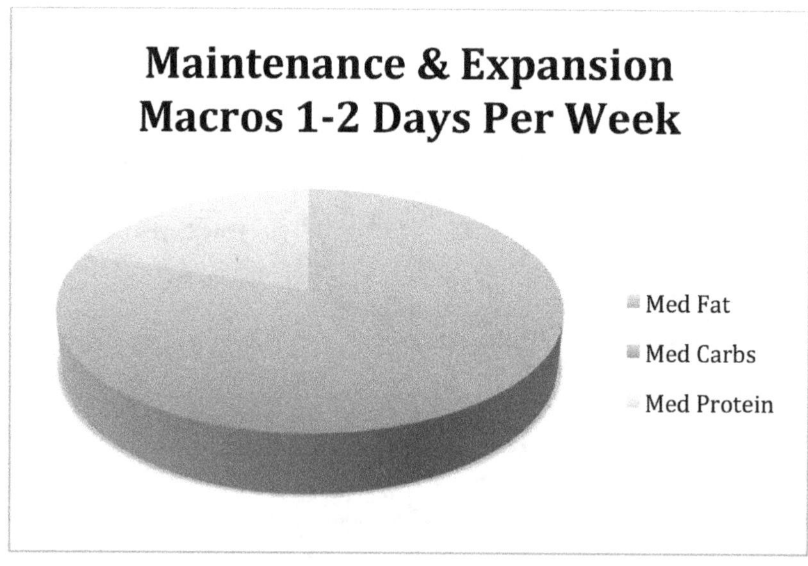

Pain Free Transition Strategies

To make this initial transition into *The Power Diet* as smooth and painless as possible you'll need to take some really important actions, so pay close attention here.

Key Action Items To Make Your Draw Down Easy!

Many people struggle with intermittent fasting simply because they don't have the right tools or strategies.

For instance, when you're detoxifying or become overwhelmed with cravings and hunger pangs, your mind may play tricks on you like telling you that you need to eat or else you'll be miserable and die.

Thankfully, when you use these transition strategies you won't fall into these traps. Eventually, by implementing these strategies for 60 days, you'll have created an irreversible habit, which you can use to create superhuman power for the rest of your life.

Accordingly, you'll need to pay special attention to the following recommendations, as they will make your lifestyle transition much more smooth and painless.

Skip Breakfast or Dinner

One of the easiest ways to stick to *The Power Diet* is to simply skip your first or last meal - breakfast or dinner.

For example, I personally do not eat breakfast 5 days a week. Instead, I just drink Yerba Mate, Matcha, Herbal Tea or Coffee potentially with a fat topper.

This gets me through the morning without the need for food but this is just what works for me personally. You may want to stop eating late night dinners or you may find that you don't need to skip any meals and can eat three smaller meals within your window. This is the beauty of *The Power Diet*; it gives you the flexibility to choose your eating window. Accordingly, I strongly encourage you to explore and see what works best for your body.

Do Not Eat 3 Hours Before Bedtime

According to studies, eating before bed can create GERD (heartburn) and nightmares, which interfere with your sleep.[179]

Additional studies show compromised sleep (less than 7-8 hours) exacerbates hunger and cravings, which makes routine tasks difficult.[180] And if this doesn't curb your late night munchies maybe this next study will.

In a 12-week study, participants who ate 50 percent of their calories at breakfast experienced more than twice the amount of weight loss compared to participants who ate 50% of their calories for dinner. Early eaters also stuck to the diet longer and showed improvements in triglyceride, cholesterol, and insulin levels throughout the day.[181]

Not eating late is a game changer and can not only help you sleep better but make you more productive. Make sure you refrain from late night food and instead focus on doing something more creative. If you have challenges with discipline and eat for emotional reasons like loneliness or boredom I recommend checking out <u>The Winner's Mindset</u>.

Drink Lots Of Liquids

Drinking sufficient liquid throughout the day is also a key player in flushing out toxins and restoring your full power. According to doctors and health professionals like Amy Hess-Fischl, RD, CDE, of the University of Chicago Kovler Diabetes Center:

"If your body does not have sufficient water, then metabolic wastes will not be removed as efficiently as they should."

Since your kidneys use water to transport toxins out of your body (primarily through sweat and urine), you should drink healthy amounts of water with natural electrolytes during your fasting window.

Specifically, during the first 30 days of employing *The Power Diet* **drink more water than you normally drink**. Once you've finished the cleansing phase and don't have headaches and flu like symptoms you can reduce your water intake to normal proportions.

This will come in huge when your hormone ghrelin starts growling for food after a couple hours of fasting in the morning. When you do get the grumbles, just know, you won't die if you don't eat. So instead of reaching for a snack or some carbo laden crack, just drink some herbal tea or spring water with lemon, lime or trace minerals.

As mentioned earlier, current recommendations for normal water consumption are .5 to 1 ounce per pound of body weight. For example, if you weighed 150 pounds, normal consumption would be somewhere between 10 and 20 cups of water (8 ounces = 1 cup).

Drink Mild Stimulants (Coffee, Green Tea or Yerba Mate)

Until you become fat adapted you will be low on energy. If you find you simply cannot concentrate I highly recommend drinking high quality, organic coffee, green tea, matcha or yerba mate during any morning fasting window.

Optionally, since butter and MCT oil do not have a major impact on the negation of ketosis you can add a teaspoon of MCT oil, raw butter, ghee or pasteurized grass fed butter to your tea or coffee. This will give you additional ketones to power your brain and prevent brain fog during your fasting periods.

Make absolutely sure you do not purchase low quality beverages, which may contain mold toxins and drain your power. See our resources page for recommendations:

www.ChadScottCoaching.com/resources

WARNING: Caffeinated beverages are acidic, can tax your adrenal glands and kill your power. Unless you want to do the jitterbug or climb walls during your fasting window keep these to 1 – 2 cups maximum per day and do not drink caffeine past 2 pm.

Get Fired Up

This may not be so obvious but when you are fasting you can absolutely engage in the recommended exercises of the *Fired Up* program. In fact, according to most experts like Mark Sisson and Dr. Joseph Mercola, conducting fasted workouts helps accelerate the process of fat adaptation, mitochondrial biogenesis (building new mitochondria) and autophagy.

Just keep in mind, if you do exercise in a fasted state and you are not yet fully fat adapted, you'll need to workout earlier in the fasting phase (between 10-14 hours).

For example, if you stopped eating at 8 pm and worked out the next morning at 8 am this would be 12 hours in a fasted state.

To test your metabolic flexibility (ability to burn fat) notice how you feel right after you workout. If you feel like you need to eat you're most likely still in the process of transitioning from stick burner to log burner. If this is the case, give yourself another month on *The Power Diet* and retest.

Once you feel like you don't need to eat right after a workout, you're burning logs my friend – congratulations! At this point, you can increase your fasting time and workout even later in your fast.

Additionally, you can wait an hour or two after working out to eat, which according to Sisson creates a flood of adaptive hormones while autophagy kicks in big time.

If this sounds interesting you can find out more about "Fired Up" here: www.ChadScottCoaching.com/fired-up

Bomb The Bugs and Feed Your Forest

When you transition from being dependent on carbs to becoming metabolically flexible, you'll be met with some resistance from those invaders and gang members we talked about earlier. In addition to reactive lectins, this includes viruses, parasites and fungi like candida that live on those carbs and sugar you've been so generously feeding them.

Unfortunately, when they are no longer being fed carbs and you lack the protection of healthy gut flora, they disrupt your microbiome and burn down your delicate forest.

So in the next chapter "Supplements", I'll recommend the most powerful herbs and supplements to effectively bomb the bad guys and rebuild your forest.

Take Hot Baths With Clay

If you have itchy spots, headaches, are battling a virus or just experience general cleansing reactions, a hot bath with clay for 30-60 minutes 2-3 days a week will work wonders. When I was battling COVID this was one of my biggest guns to counterattack the virus.

Effectively, a hot bath or sauna has been proven to stop the replication of a virus dead in its tracks by inducing a fever. This is your body's natural reaction to burn out unwanted invaders and it's also the reason why you get a natural fever when you get the flu.

According to Dr. James DiNicolantonio, the Associate Editor of Nutrition and British Medical Journal's (BMJ) Open Heart, high heat exposure activates heat shock proteins, which may prevent viral nucleoproteins from being exported suppressing viral replication.

For example, a clinical study involving 50 volunteers showed regular sauna bathers had half the rate of common cold compared to nonusers. Doctors like DiNicolantonio and Joe Mercola believe this could be a highly effective tool in beating a virus like COVID-19, especially if employed prior or early on in infection.[182]

And when it comes to detoxification and the "keto flu" a hot bath or steam also induces a fever and allows your body to sweat out many toxins. Additionally, by adding a certain type of clay with minerals you can neutralize toxins and bring rapid relief.

Personally, even though I eat a clean diet and exercise regularly, I still absorb enough toxins from my environment (smog, chemicals, etc.) to justify taking a hot bath two nights a week and I can't recommend it enough.   Since this is so important I've outlined some guidelines for hot baths as follows:

- **Ideal Temperature** - Since hot water can break down your skin's protective barrier, which guards against pollution, germs, and bacteria, make sure your bath is between 96 to 104 degrees. If you do not have a thermometer dip your hand it. If it's too hot to hold your hand in for more than a few seconds, let it cool down until you can hold your hand in for a few seconds without too much discomfort.

- **Ideal Time** - While the amount of time needed to detoxify is widely debated, the hotter your bath water is the quicker you'll be detoxifying and the less time you'll need to stay in the bath. I recommend basing your time in the bath on your time available. For example, I don't have a lot of time to spare so I turn the heat up close to 104 and spend about 15-30 minutes. When I get out I'm sweating for an additional 30 minutes, which gives me a powerful detox effect. If you have more time you can simply turn the heat down and spend up to 1 hour.

- **Music & Learning** - Lastly, in order to optimize your time in the bath, I recommend listening to something on your smartphone. If you feel like your brain has been working overtime and you have a lot of stress I recommend listening to some relaxing music for a more meditative experience. In contrast, if your brain is not overworked, I recommend listening to a fiction or non-fiction audiobook. For recommendations on clay or any of these supplements check out our resources page at:

www.ChadScottCoaching.com/resources.

Power Supplements

Congratulations! If you've gotten to this point you're more than likely moving forward on *The Power Diet*, eating amazing meals and working towards burning logs and feeling powerful.

Sadly, no matter how much power boosting food you eat or how much power draining food you eliminate, it's just not going to be enough to supply the vital nutrients you need for optimal health and maximum power. There are several reasons for this dilemma, the first of which is soil depletion.

Essentially, the earth in which food is grown, which feeds us humans and the plants and animals we eat, has been depleted of valuable micronutrients, vitamins and minerals. This, in turn, has a direct effect on the quality of the foods we consume on a regular basis organic or otherwise.

Secondly, research is now showing that as you age you lose the ability to produce various power boosters like testosterone, NAD+ and CoQ10. And unless you live near the equator and get lots of sun exposure you're probably also deficient in vitamin D, one of nature's greatest superpowers.

Thirdly, if you contract a virus like COVID-19 or any other illness you'll want to actively institute a counterattack and wipe out that invader as soon as possible with mother natures power supplements.

To be clear, I don't have a supplement company. My goal here is to simply recommend the most important supplements, which will boost your fighting power and shore up any cracks in your diet as you sail off toward your island full of treasure.

Make no mistake about it; these supplements can be game changers, so I recommend investing what you can afford and experimenting with the options provided.

Speaking of which, you'll find two main categories "Daily" and "Occasional." The daily supplements are divided into two sub-categories, "Nutritional Supplements" and "Anti-aging Supplements." These can be taken daily to plug nutritional gaps and slow the aging process.

"Occasional" supplements includes two additional sub-categories "Anti-viral Supplements" and "Power Supplements" that should be taken on occasion, i.e. during the cold and flu season, when you get sick or when you want to increase your workout performance or lift your libido.

Make sure you keep experimenting until you find your own personal sweet spot of optimized performance.

Top Nutritional Supplements

First up in daily recommendations are my top nutritional supplements. This is not an exhaustive list; rather, these are simply the most important which have been shown through studies to be low in the majority of the population. These will function to shore up any nutritional deficiencies from your diet. If for any reason you don't have the budget for all of them just buy what you can by starting with #1.

Daily Supplements

#1 - Krill Oil / Spirulina / Algae Oil

EPA and DHA are known as omega-3 fatty acids, which your body cannot produce, which is why they are also known as "essential" fatty acids. Sadly, studies show that the average person's diet only provides 10% of the EPA and DHA needed to preserve health and prevent disease.[183]

Further studies show that insufficient EPA and DHA intake can increase the risk of a number of health conditions, including heart disease, Alzheimer's, and cancer.[184]

Naturally, there's a massive benefit to increasing your EPA and DHA and why most health experts recommend it as the #1 most important supplement. Studies show it can boost your life on many fronts including:

- Improve your mood and decrease depression, anxiety, and stress.[185]

- Increase cognitive performance, with better memory recall, longer attention span, and quicker reaction time.[186]
- Reduced muscle and joint soreness.[187]
- Improve fat loss.[188]
- Prevent fat gain.[189]
- Gain muscle faster.[190]

While the most obvious power foods for EPA and DHA are fish you can also get this potent ingredient in grass-fed meat, free-range eggs, and vegetable oils. Unfortunately, unless you eat truckloads of them every day, you're not going to get the quantity needed for optimal health or maximum power. This is where Krill Oil comes in big! As Dr. Joe Mercola explains:

"Krill oil carries omega-3s in the form of phospholipids, little packages that deliver fatty acids across your cellular membranes directly to your body's cells… Scientific evidence to date has shown that the safest and most effective carriers of EPA and DHA are these phospholipids."

But that's not all as Krill oil is jam-packed with antioxidant power. If you're not already familiar with antioxidants, these are compounds that inhibit oxidation. Similar to rust on iron, oxidation is a chemical reaction that can produce free radicals, thereby leading to chain reactions that may damage the cells of organisms.

While antioxidants such as Vitamin C can terminate these chain reactions, krill oil contains Astaxanthin, one of the most powerful antioxidants on the planet, which is 6,000 times stronger than vitamin C, 800 times stronger than CoQ10, 550 times stronger than Green Tea Catechins and 75 times stronger than Alpha Lipoic Acid. Not only that but krill oil also contains vitamins A and E, two more powerful antioxidants necessary for optimum health.

Vegetarians/Vegans - If you eat very little or no fish and animal products, there's a really good chance you'll be low on protein, vitamin B12 and Omega-3 fats, which can drain your power significantly.

If this is you, I recommend taking either a spirulina or an algae oil supplement daily. Ironically, the reason why fish and shellfish have so much beneficial omega-3 is because they eat algae. You can bypass the middleman (fish and shellfish) and go straight to the source of omega-3 fats if this seems like a more practical solution for your particular circumstances.

Check out our resources page for the best and most trusted recommendations here: www.ChadScottCoaching.com.

#2 - Rebuild Your Forest With Probiotics & Prebiotics

As stated at the beginning of *The Power Diet*, your gut wall contains 70% of your immune power and once this is compromised all hell breaks loose. So in addition to avoiding toxins, eating fermented foods and bombing the bad guys, you'll need to rebuild your forest with both probiotics and prebiotics.

Probiotics are 'good' bacteria that line your digestive tract and support your body's ability to digest and assimilate nutrients, support immunity and fight infections, regulate weight and even balance hormones.

Remember, it's not just calories that create weight gain but hormones and studies show that probiotics can help you lose unwanted weight by balancing hormones.[191]

Prebiotics, on the other hand are the food, which feeds your healthy bacteria and supports a long-term strategy for rebuilding your microbiome. Some of the power foods mentioned earlier are considered prebiotics like jicama, garlic, onions, cabbage, chicory root, radish and artichokes.

While you can get both probiotics and prebiotics from food it's just not going to be enough to regrow a fully powered microbiome. As such, I recommend taking a combination supplement of these for 3-4 months, then cycling off for 30 days to make sure your gut doesn't become desensitized to an overabundance of the same flora.

After a 30-day break, you can either continue the cycle by reintroducing the same bacteria or try another formula to give your gut flora more diversity.

While you could buy prebiotics and probiotics separately I recommend one of the most trusted and potent brands, which contains both. Check out our resources page for the best and most trusted recommendations here: www.ChadScottCoaching.com.

#3 - Whole-Food Vitamins and Minerals

A number of carefully controlled studies provide startling evidence that by the time processed food reaches your table serious nutrient content could already be lost; in some cases over 50 percent!

For example, a 2004 study evaluated Department of Agriculture data for 43 garden crops from 1950 to 1999 and found statistically reliable declines for six nutrients: protein, calcium, potassium, iron and vitamins B2 and C.[192]

Fortunately, with a good whole food based multi, you'll get around 50 whole food based vitamins and minerals to fill the nutritional gap. This includes powerhouses like magnesium, which plays a role in hundreds of enzymatic bodily reactions, like metabolizing food, synthesizing fatty acids and proteins, and transmission of nerve impulses so you don't get leg cramps in the middle of the night.

Of course, this is just one of many nutrients and doesn't account for perhaps one of the biggest power players – Vitamin D.

Nearly every cell in your body, including your heart, brain, and even fat cells, uses this essential nutrient and studies show it regulates genes that control immune function, metabolism, and even cell growth and development. [193]

This is highly significant since insufficient vitamin D levels have been shown to be associated with an increased risk of many types of disease, including osteoporosis, heart disease, stroke, some cancers, type 1 diabetes, multiple sclerosis, tuberculosis, and even the flu virus.[194]

And if you have any gut issues as I did, Vitamin D3 helps heal your gut lining from all those reactive lectin bombs you've most likely been eating all your life.

Unfortunately, our bodies have a difficult time producing enough vitamin D to maintain adequate levels and fight off disease, so we must obtain it from our diet, sun exposure, or supplementation.[195]

While I recommend a good multi with a dose of 2,000 – 4,000 IUs of D3 daily (it's more effective than D2), if you do not get much sun exposure, have leaky gut, digestive issues, or do not eat eggs and fish I highly recommend getting a separate Vitamin D supplement and using between 4,000 IUs to about 10,000 IUs per day. Interestingly, this has been shown to provide a significant and beneficial effect on measures of exercise performance.[196] [197]

Similarly, if you have immune challenges you may need a more therapeutic dosage of vitamin C with a specific type called liposomal. We'll talk more about that in the Immunity boosters shortly.

If you have problems sleeping or experience restless leg syndrome you may also want to buy a separate magnesium supplement, which will allow you to take a more therapeutic dosage.

Just keep in mind; a good multi should contain your key vitamins like C, B3, B12, and D3 plus essential minerals like magnesium, copper, iron and calcium.

Considering the critical depletion of soil nutrients combined with all the toxins in our environment and the difficult access to clean organic foods, hopefully, it's becoming clear why you need to add a good multivitamin to plug any holes in your diet.

Lastly, it's important to understand that a multivitamin has fat-soluble Vitamins like A, D, E and K, which should be taken with food that contains fat, which obviously shouldn't be much of a problem if your taking it with a power diet meal. Check out our resources page for the best and most trusted recommendations here: www.ChadScottCoaching.com.

Top Anti-aging Supplements

#1 - CoQ10 / Ubiquinol

According to most experts like Dr. Mercola, one of the key elements in the aging process is free radical production, which we've talked about on several occasions.

Free radicals cause damage to your tissues and DNA. Therefore, it stands to reason, if you can limit free radical production, you can potentially influence the normal aging process by slowing it down if not reversing it completely.

Other than keeping your blood glucose levels low by lowering carb and protein consumption, by adding one of Mother Nature's powerhouse nutrients, CoQ10, or its active, reduced form, Ubiquinol you can boost the life extension functions of *The Power Diet*.

Effectively, your body requires the reduced form of CoQ10 (ubiquinol) to help you limit free radical production. And as you age, it becomes more and more difficult to convert the oxidized CoQ10 to ubiquinol. This power booster has some remarkable effects including:

- Boosts your body's cellular energy production and supports the health of your cells' mitochondria that produce nearly all of your body's energy.

- Helps facilitate the production of adenosine triphosphate (ATP), the energy "currency" for all your cells.

- Enables a strong first stage defense against oxygen free radicals to help you reduce the signs of premature aging.

If you are under 30 years old you can benefit from CoQ10 but if you're over 30 you'll need the reduced form of CoQ10, Ubiquinol, to efficiently carry out all of its functions. Check out our resources page for the best and most trusted recommendations here: www.ChadScottCoaching.com.

#2 NAD+ Power Restoration

All the amazing foods from *The Power Diet* won't do much good if your cells can't extract energy from them. Fortunately, under the right conditions, our bodies naturally produce Nicotinamide adenine dinucleotide, or NAD, a coenzyme found in every cell, which is crucial to the basic reactions in your cells that keep you alive.

NAD occurs in two forms: NAD+ and NADH and according to Harvard Medical School professor "Dr. David Sinclair" is:

"The closest we've gotten to a fountain of youth."

The two power players NAD+ and NADH are responsible for a host of life lifting abilities including:

Anti-Aging - As an anti-aging mechanism they keep your telomeres working efficiently and according to New York Times bestseller of "The Telomere Effect," Dr. Elissa Epel:

"When we measure telomeres in midlife, they're a pretty reliable predictor of who gets disease early and, in some studies, who dies early. So, they do matter when we're older."

And if you're not already hip to this term "telomere" it relates directly to how long or short you will live and NAD+ has shown in multiple studies to help protect your cells from age related decline and help lengthen your lifespan.[198] [199]

More Energy – NAD helps with the conversion of protein, fat, and carbohydrate into energy - obviously important if you want more power.[200] [201]

Stress Reduction – Multiple studies show that NAD+ makes your cells more resilient to stress, which as you now know is a major power drain.[202] [203]

Sleep Well & Eat Right - Studies have identified the role of NAD+ in sleep cycles and hunger patterns and by upping your production you can sleep deeper and stop eating at the wrong times.[204] [205] [206]

DNA Repair – DNA is the foundation of your basic cell structure and once it's damaged you start to go downhill.

Fortunately, NAD+ facilitates DNA repair to aging body parts.[207]

Of course, with such incredible potential for expanded power this begs the question: How do you get more NAD+?

Well, there's some good news and even more good news here. Fortunately, *The Power Diet* has built in NAD+ boosting strategies.

Specifically, by following the 2nd Pillar "Quantity" or eating the right macros (50-70% fat) your body will go into ketosis and automatically increases the NAD+ to NADH ratio. This is important since the science shows we need higher NAD+ because it protects cells from oxidative stress.[208][209]

Secondly, by following the 3rd Pillar "Frequency" or intermittent fasting, the science also shows you'll be naturally boosting your NAD+ levels.[210][211]

And while following *The Power Diet* will boost your NAD+ levels significantly, as you age, other chemical processes kick in and your natural production starts to decline.[212] For this reason, I recommend trying an NAD+ supplement and noticing if you get a boost in overall power.

Again, there are loads of fake products out there so I recommend checking out our resources section for a good recommendation.

Occasional Supplements

As mentioned previously, occasional supplements are divided into two sub-categories: "Anti-Viral Boosters" needed during the cold and flu season and "Power Boosters" when you need a boost of power or a lift in libido. Let's go ahead and investigate how these can improve your life.

Anti-Viral Boosters

With the outbreak of new viruses like COVID-19 we now live in the age of super-bugs. And while *The Power Diet* and *Fired Up* program will function as your primary line of defense, by adding in some super powered supplements you can turbo charge your immune system and prevent or fight off the invaders with much greater ease.

#1 – Antioxidants & Polyphenols

If you're sick or under constant threat of getting sick during the winter or during a pandemic like COVID-19 you'll want to remain slightly alkaline as much as possible. Remember, your power and immunity is directly related to your pH level and when you become too acidic you become an easy target for invaders.

Fortunately, in addition to eating an alkaline diet like *The Power Diet* you can up your intake of Polyphenols, micronutrients from plant-based foods that are packed with antioxidants, which can boost your immunity in a big way.

For example, multiple studies show that the antioxidant Vitamin C may prevent the susceptibility of lower respiratory tract infections.[213] Additionally, many reports from China indicate patients with COVID-19 who have been administered large doses of intravenous vitamin C have, as a result, been released from critical care shortly thereafter.

Since oral vitamin C made from corn (ascorbic acid) is typically less effective than intravenous administration, due in part to inferior bioavailability, I recommend buying "Liposomal" Vitamin C, which has been proven to have a much higher absorption rate.[214]

Once you feel the onset of symptoms like headache, fever, sore throat or chills I recommend taking at least 3-5 Grams of liposomal Vitamin C three times a day until symptoms subside.

When I was dealing with COVID this made a huge difference. Additionally, I recently stepped on a bee and got stung while walking barefoot on the beach. After waking up the next day with an infection and massive boil of puss on my foot, I took 5 grams of vitamin C and the infection disappeared within 24 hours.

To boost your alkalinity under the stress of illness I recommend bone broth soups and occasional raw green drinks made mostly of vegetables. And if you don't have access to raw green drinks make sure you buy an antioxidant powder made of spirulina, greens and fruits, which you can mix in water and drink a couple times per day. Just make sure you don't buy greens with reactive lectins like grasses or barley as these may create a negative reaction.

As an added bonus to balancing your pH Level and boosting your immunity, these antioxidants, vitamins, minerals and electrolytes will speed up the cleansing process and help eliminate any flu like symptoms during your transition from carbo stick burner to fat fuel log burner.

Again, if you are uncertain about recommendations check our resources page.

#2 - Oregano Oil – Bomb The Bugs

As mentioned earlier, during your initial foray into intermittent fasting, you'll experience cravings from time to time as well as gut instability from pathogens, viruses, parasites, yeast and bacteria that feed on sugar.

To expedite the natural process of *The Power Diet* and eliminate the bad bugs and invaders you can occasionally drop a few green oregano bombs down the pipes.

Since oregano oil has been proven to be more effective than penicillin in wiping out unwanted invaders without the negative side effects, we'll be using a powerful version of it.[215]

Specifically, I recommend taking 3 oregano capsules when you start to feel cravings or when you have a gut issue from a virus or bacteria that just doesn't seem to resolve by fasting.

Since the last few hours of your fast tend to be the toughest, a good time to drop those bombs is around 1-3 hours before your fast is over.

While becoming fat adapted over time will be your main strategy for eliminating cravings for carbs, by tossing a few of these green bombs down the pipes you'll score a direct hit and silence those invaders as well as a good chunk of those carbo cravings. Do this until symptoms resolve (no more than 30 days) then cycle off.

If at some point in the future you fall off the wagon or experience the cravings and invaders again you can cycle back onto Oregano until symptoms resolve.

Just keep in mind, if you buy a low quality brand you'll have to take twice as much. Instead, I recommend purchasing the most potent and trusted brand for Oregano Oil. Check out our resources page for the best and most trusted products here: www.ChadScottCoaching.com.

#3 Elderberry with Zinc

Researchers have found compounds in the elderberry, which could directly inhibit the flu virus's entrance into cells and subsequent replication. Flu-fighting properties had been observed in previous studies, but this group examined the actual mechanism, the phytochemicals used to combat the influenza infection.[216][217]

Zinc has also been found to stop the replication of a virus including the Coronavirus and combined with vitamin C, D and Elderberry creates a powerful immune cocktail to crush just about any unwanted invader. [218][219]

If you're battling an illness I recommend taking your C, D Elderberry and Zinc separately and at least tripling the recomended dosage of all of them. While you can buy combinations of zinc and elderberry, the zinc will not be absorbed as effectively as a standalone ionic liquid zinc formula. Again, check out my resources page for the best recommendations.

Power Boosters

The following power boosters are backed by multiple studies and can be used to occasionally boost your workouts and build more strength or lift your libido when the time is right.

Maca

Maca is a sweet root vegetable related to cruciferous vegetables like broccoli, cauliflower and kale, which is found mostly in South America. While it is considered a power food, since it's unavailable in most supermarkets you'll more likely find this as supplement or dried powder, which you can add to a smoothie.

Commonly known to boost fertility, Maca is also referred to as "The Peruvian Viagra" and is one of the rare aphrodisiacs actually backed by multiple scientific studies.

For example, four respectable studies reported that participants experienced enhanced sexual desire after they consumed maca. [220] [221] [222] [223]

An additional smaller study suggests that maca may help reduce the loss of libido associated with certain side effects from antidepressant drugs. [224]

And while most studies provided 1.5–3.5 grams of maca per day for 2–12 weeks with very few side effects, [225] you'll want to experiment with your own personal tolerance level.

Creatine – Fast Track To Results

As one of the safest, most well researched organic compounds in all of sports nutrition, Creatine helps you get stronger and build muscle faster while improving anaerobic performance and reducing recovery time. [226] [227] [228] [229] [230]

What's the secret weapon behind this power player?

Composed of the amino acids, L-arginine, glycine, and L-methionine, Creatine is an organic compound, which can be found in most of the same foods as Vitamin D like meat, eggs, and fish.

What's interesting about Creatine is that it's present in almost all cells, where it acts as an "energy reserve." So when you take a supplement of this power player, your total body Creatine stores increase, with most going to your muscle cells. [231]

Of course, when your muscle cells have more energy your performance goes up. But perhaps even cooler is how this positively affects nitrogen and the expression of certain genes related to muscle building. [232]

If this sounds appealing make sure you go with a product that has high standards and won't upset your stomach. Specifically, you'll need powdered Creatine monohydrate, which has been researched and tested for efficacy and safety. Check out our resources page for the best and most trusted recommendations here: www.ChadScottCoaching.com.

L-Citrulline / L-Arginine

L-citrulline is an amino acid made by your body and contained in certain foods, which is converted by your body into another type of amino acid L-arginine.

If you're in the fitness world or read the trades you may have noticed the popularity of these amino acids, and for good reason. Several studies show they can significantly improve both resistance and endurance training.

For example, in one study, scientists from the University of Cordoba demonstrated how supplementation with 8 grams of L-citrulline before a chest workout increased the number of reps participants could do by 52 percent with an added bonus of significantly reducing post workout muscle soreness.[233]

But What Is It That Provides The Boost Of Power?

Unsurprisingly, it's none other than that highly coveted secret agent of libido boosting power - nitric oxide. Yes, L-citrulline, which is converted to L-arginine produces significant quantities of nitric oxide and nitric oxide increases blood flow to your sexual organs! [234]

How To Get L-Citrulline

L-citrulline is most abundant in foods like meat and nuts. Quite ironic when you think about how this relates to your thriving sex organs once you bone up on L-Citrulline.

But that's not all! Several foods contain L-citrulline so I've created a shortlist of foods that should be on your plate daily.

Meat   - preferably organic and grass-fed
Fish   - preferably wild caught low mercury
Nuts   - preferably skinless almonds and walnuts
Onion - preferably organic
Garlic - preferably organic

While you should be eating these foods daily, in order to recreate those studies and get enough nitric oxide to boost your libido you're most likely going to need to take a supplement. When you look online you'll find hundreds of choices but again, quality is really important here as fake products with fillers are the norm, not the exception.

How Much Should I Take?

The second thing you'll need to consider is the dosage. While I do recommend starting with the "recommended dosage" on the label, you'll need to experiment and see what your body can tolerate. If you do not have any risk of heart disease I recommend ramping up towards 8 -10 grams per day until you notice a boost in power.

There are not many long-term studies on supplementation so I would not take this every day. Instead, rely on your meat and nuts and supplement once in a while when you need a power boost.

While you can take this in pill or powder form I recommend trying "Doctors Best" powder and adding it to water or a smoothie. It's virtually tasteless and odorless so you don't have to worry about what you take it with. Check out our resources section for recommendations at:

www.ChadScottCoaching.com/resources

Supplement Quantity And Frequency

It's important to understand that the three elements of quality, quantity and frequency also apply to your supplements, so let's get clear on what to look for.

Supplement Quality

When it comes to supplement quality you want to avoid synthetic power drains and instead opt for "Whole Food Based" supplements. The supplement should be derived directly from a food source and in most cases say: "Whole Food" somewhere on the packaging.

Secondly, you should always buy from a reputable source that has great reviews. If you are uncertain check out my recommendations at http://www.ChadScottCoaching.com/

Quantity & Frequency

How much you take and how often you take it should be outlined in the manufacturer's recommended dosage.

There are exceptions though. For instance, to reproduce the effects of a particular study like the ones we just mentioned from ginseng you'll need to take the dosage used in the study. Just make sure you read the label and back off if you feel anything unusual or painful.

The Grand Finale

And now, we've come to the end, the grand finale! This is where we tie everything together and make *The Power Diet* super simple to remember.

To recap, there are three main pillars of *The Power Diet* – Quality, Quantity and Frequency! If you can remember these when you buy food and you eat it you'll transform your life in ways you never thought possible, with more energy, productivity, power, strength, less sick days and more feel good days.

To make this super simple I've created "**The Power Diet Master Guide**," which is a downloadable reference chart you can use to stay on track and build your power.

While I recommend re-reading this book several times to really retain the information, by downloading this guide you'll be able to quickly build meals from the 5 power food categories and begin forming the eating habits that will bulletproof your immunity and build your power for the rest of your life!

Take Action – Get Started Now!

Remember, without action, you simply won't get any new results. Make sure you take action right now and get started by following these action steps.

Step 1) Download *The Power Diet Master Guide*. Go ahead do that now then do two things with it:

a) Download it to your smartphone and reference it when you shop, cook or order food!

Download: https://chadscottcoaching.com/PD-Master-G.jpg

b) Print and/or laminate it and put it on your refrigerator! Any local print shop can laminate your guide for a couple dollars so you can attach it to your refrigerator with a magnet.

Step 2) Clear Out The Power Drains

Before you begin *The Power Diet*, you'll need to get rid of the temptations that drain your power. This means clearing out the power drains from your refrigerator, kitchen cabinets, car, office, purse, pockets, backpacks or anywhere else you keep those carbo laden toxic treats.

If you recoil at the thought of throwing stuff away, just think about all the money you'll save in the long run by not getting cancer and going through chemotherapy or not getting heart disease and having to take prescription drugs for the rest of your life.

And let's not forget about bypassing diabetes and having to take shots of insulin for the rest of your life. Oh yeah, did I mention dodging the lifeless, depressing sugar crash from eating more toxic food?

Now is the time to get really serious. This is your life we're talking about and it's more valuable than a bag of potato chips, a candy bar, soda pop or a slice of bread. Your body is your temple; it's the vehicle that will carry you through this life and make your dreams a reality.

On the flip side, if you do not take action I can guarantee you'll regret it at the end of your life (remember our study from the top regrets of the dying?).

Think of your mind and body like a fine tuned Ferrari; they both need high-octane fuel and when you dump low-grade fuel like Coke, McDonalds or a bunch of wheat bread in it, things start to shut down and eventually it blows up.

The Ultimate Comeback Line

Once you become a log burner you'll experience criticism from people who say you're no fun because you don't slog down Slurpees and stuff yourself full of toxic treats.

If you find someone tries to pull you down, first, express compassion and just know that they haven't been able to step up like you have. This may be intimidating to them so they react by attempting to bring you down so they can feel good about themselves.

Second, you can comeback with a sharp and witty line that will baffle even the most cynical of beings with this:

You can't put a bag of sugar in a Ferrari!

Of course, you can swap out bag of sugar with whatever the debate is about. Either way, I guarantee they'll be thinking twice about making fun of you for having the discipline to limit or eliminate toxic treats and who knows, maybe you'll inspire them to step their game up and advance their own health.

Now go ahead and grab a garbage bag, make a sweep of all your stashes and take it out to the trash. Don't even think twice about keeping it or giving it to someone else who also doesn't need it.

Throw it away and say: Thank God… I'm finally going to be free of the chains of toxic food. It's liberation time, baby!

Next, after you've thrown all the temptations away, you're going to need to set a goal.

Step 3) Set A Non-Negotiable Goal

If for any reason you believe goals are a waste of time, you may as well just throw in the towel and give up now.

Really, if you just think about all the times you told yourself or someone else you needed to take action on something important and never followed through I'd wager you'd be able to recall at least a few missed opportunities.

The real question here is why didn't you take action? Could it be that you simply didn't believe it was that important and you were not fully committed to take the action necessary to make it happen?

Unfortunately, as we mentioned at the start of this book, without action your desires and goals are just dreams you'll take with you to the grave. But when you set a "Non-Negotiable" goal by writing it down, sharing it with others and scheduling it in your calendar, you'll have a much better chance at achieving that goal.

So think of this non-negotiable goal as an unbreakable pact with yourself; something that you must do or else your entire life will be a complete waste of time.

For instance, would you have any regrets if you made food more important than anything else in your life and as a result died overweight at an early age, instead of cultivating loving relationships with your family or working on your dreams?

Would you have any regrets if you spent your whole life as a carb junky, a prisoner, who constantly had to eat matchstick food that created inflammation, which eventually killed you with a fatal heart disease?

Now just take a minute to re-read those two scenarios and really feel the pain of regret. This is really important because it helps you get leverage over the weak minded carb junky that isn't willing to take the action necessary to really step up and set yourself free.

Next, after you've read those scenarios and really felt how important it is to take control of your health do you now feel a stronger commitment to taking action on *The Power Diet*?

I'm going to assume that's a big "Yes," which means it's time to get serious and feed your Ferrari with some high-octane fuel. To do this you'll need to ask yourself the following question:

What do I need most when it comes to food?

There are typically two obvious goals here. The first of which is to simply lose weight. If this is you, you'll want to set a goal to lose 50% of your target weight loss within 1-3 months and the other 50% in another 1-3 months.

So let's say you're 50 pounds overweight and you set a goal to lose 25 pounds in 3 months with an additional 25 pounds in another 3 months. Since 50 pounds is a good chunk of fat and losing too much weight too quickly (more than 2 pounds per week) can could put you at risk of many health problems, including muscle loss, gallstones and nutritional deficiencies, this goal can realistically be achieved by simply sticking to *The Power Diet*. [235] [236]

In contrast, if you are 20 pounds overweight you could more easily create a goal of losing 10 pounds in 1-2 months and an additional 10 pounds in another 1-2 months.

The next most common goal I find is to simply increase power and feel great or solve a health issue like leaky gut, insulin resistance or arthritis. If this is you, I recommend setting your goal to get through the 8-week drawdown period and become a full-fledged member of the log burner club.

To get clear on what a non-negotiable goal would look like for you let's take a look at a few examples:

Weight Loss

I am committed to losing 16 pounds in 8 weeks and will take all the action steps in *The Power Diet* by scheduling them in my calendar and following through. Taking these actions is non-negotiable! I am 100% committed to my health and will not break my pact with myself no matter what the circumstances are!

Health Issue

I am committed to getting rid of my stomach pain and will take all the action steps in *The Power Diet* by scheduling them in my calendar and following through. Taking these actions is non-negotiable! I am 100% committed to my health and will not break my pact with myself no matter what the circumstances are!

Feeling Better with More Power

I am committed to feeling better with more power and energy. I will take all the action steps in *The Power Diet* by scheduling them in my calendar and following through. Taking these actions is non-negotiable! I am 100% committed to my health and will not break my pact with myself no matter what the circumstances are!

NOTE: While that 100% commitment statement at the end may sound a bit rigid, just remember *The Power Diet* is not rigid, it's flexible and allows you to have fun, enjoy food and splurge once in a while. The commitment here is simply to stick to "The Three Pillars" of *The Power Diet*.

Write Down Your Non-Negotiable Goal Now!

Now go ahead and take action by writing down your non-negotiable goal and placing it somewhere you can see it every day like your kitchen or bathroom. I suggest printing this out and framing it in a plastic frame like this one <u>from Amazon</u>, which only costs a few dollars.

Step 4) – Get Accountability & Support

Taking action on the first three steps is a great start but you'll need to take one more crucial step if you are to fully commit and take the necessary action to create a lifetime habit. This brings us to the final piece of the commitment puzzle: accountability! As personal development master Jim Rohn once said:

> ***"You are the average of the five people***
> ***you spend the most time with?"***

Adding to this wise perspective is Jim's most successful mentee Tony Robbins who declared:

> ***"Most people's lives are a direct reflection of***
> ***the expectations of their peer group."***

Yes, you'll need to make an effort to surround yourself with people who are also trying to improve themselves or in the business of self-improvement. And if you're at all doubtful of this advice consider the following study conducted by The American Society of Training and Development (ASTD).

In this study, researchers found that you have a 65% chance of completing a goal if you commit to someone.

Additionally, if you have a specific accountability appointment with a person you've committed, you will increase your chance of success by up to 95%.[237]

To stay on track and push through the inevitable minefields along the way, you'll need to actively seek out people to surround yourself with who are trying to improve their health or are interested in your health. These people, which could also be coaches, teachers, and mentors, will help you stay on track by supporting you with encouragement, experience and knowledge no single teacher could ever provide.

They'll also help in holding you accountable, which will give you a much needed push when you lose motivation and things seem hopeless.

Let's face it; in the beginning, when you're excited about feeling good, you'll probably take some action for the first few weeks. But four, five or ten weeks down the road, if you don't have the motivation, discipline and accountability to stay on track, you may just sink into a comfortable couch and gorge yourself on power draining foods.

To avoid this trap, right now you'll need to take action by finding an accountability partner. Go ahead and **call or text someone** who cares about your health and tell them about your non-negotiable goal.

We'll talk more about accountability in a moment but for now, this is the simplest thing you can do to get accountability.

Text or Call your accountability partner now!

Step 5) The Next Level

If you have any questions or challenges implementing *The Power Diet* and making it a long-term lifestyle just know, I got your back!

If for any reason you feel challenged to implement these action steps or feel like your level of discipline just can't support the transformation, I'd like to invite you to check out my intelligent accountability coaching and online trainings for boosting your brain and body to maximum power and living up to your full potential.

This includes *Fired Up*, a supercharged fitness program that combines the power and synergy of strength training, yoga and high intensity interval training. *Fired Up* is the companion program to *The Power Diet* and works synergistically to accelerate the building of a powerful, strong, and flexible mind and body. You can find out more info on this program by following this link:

Fired Up - Unleash Your Super Human Power

If you struggle with discipline and taking action I recommend one of the most powerful brain building programs ever created called "The Winner's Mindset."

This powerful audio program uses advanced neurological repatterning techniques to help you embed the mindsets of over 175 masters from sports, business, politics, arts, science, medicine and spirituality.

The Winner's Mindset took me over 10 years to create and it's my most trusted source for guaranteed results in all areas of life including increasing your wealth, finding love, building relationships and boosting your health. To find out more visit the following link:

The Winner's Mindset

With that, I'd like close with my best go to recipes and congratulate you. You're now well on your way to building a habit that will support your health and boost your power for the rest of your life. Just make absolutely sure you take action on those top 5 steps just mentioned. If you can do that I guarantee you will see success.

Wishing you the best on your journey.

Chad Scott

Power Diet Recipes

While I encourage a diverse diet with lots of power foods, in reality, most people gravitate towards a few favorite dishes. With this in mind, I've provided recipes for my six most popular dishes. Feel free to modify these recipes depending on what you find in your local stores, just make sure you try to add ingredients from the five categories mentioned previously.

Additionally, I've also included my three most popular smoothies, which can be eaten as a full meal replacement for breakfast, lunch or dinner. Enjoy!

Coconut Curry Power Bowl

Ingredients for 1 Serving

Category 1) Raw Veggies

1. *Baby Romaine Lettuce (or other lettuce) - handful*
2. *Watermelon Radish (or red radish)*
3. *Carrot - 1*
4. *Sea Salt - a couple pinches or 1/2 teaspoon*
5. *Curry Spice*
6. *Raw honey - 1 teaspoon*
7. *Lime - 1/2*
8. *Optional - Avocado - 1/2*
9. *Optional - Ginger - 1 tablespoon*

Category 1) Steamed Veggies

1. *Cauliflower - 1/2 cup*
2. *Bok Choy - 1/2 cup*
3. *Asparagus - 1/3 cup chopped*

Category 2) Coconut Oil (optional: walnut or olive oil) 1-2 tablespoons

Category 3) Sliced (blanched) Almonds 1-2 tablespoons

Category 4) Starch - Sweet potato 1/4 cup chopped

Category 5) Protein - Wild Caught Salmon (or Chicken, Beef or Vegan Hemp Tofu) 2-3 oz.

Preparation

1. Chop and dice cauliflower, asparagus and sweet potato then put in steamer for 10 minutes.   If your fish or protein is frozen put it in with these items, otherwise wait until the last 3 minutes.
2. Prepare salad with lettuce, sliced radishes, carrots and put in bowl
3. Prepare sauce with oil, nuts, salt (Note: coconut oil must be heated lightly to turn into liquid)
4. Spread steamed veggies on salad, then top with protein, then with optional avocado.
5. Top off all ingredients with sauce, and then squeeze lime on top.

Asian Power Bowl

Ingredients for 1 Serving

Category 1) Raw Veggies

1. *Butterleaf Lettuce (or other lettuce) - handful*
2. *Radicchio - 1/4 cup*
3. *Watermelon Radish (or red radish)*
4. *Avocado - 1/2*
5. *Ginger - 1 tablespoon chopped (or 1/2 teaspoon of powder)*
6. *Apple cider vinegar (or lemon) 1 tablespoon*
7. *Sea Salt - a couple pinches or 1/2 teaspoon*
8. *Optional Coconut Aminos - 1 tablespoon*

Category 1) Steamed Veggies

1. *Cauliflower - 1/2 cup*
2. *Broccoli - 1/2 cup*

Category 2) Coconut Oil (optional: walnut or olive oil) 1-2 tablespoons

Category 3) Walnuts and Tahini butter (Option: Sliced (blanched) Almonds) 1-2 tablespoons

Category 4) Starch - Sweet potato - 1/4 cup chopped

Category 5) Protein - Wild Caught Shrimp (or Chicken, Fish, Beef or Vegan Hemp Tofu) 2-3 oz.

Preparation

1. Chop and dice cauliflower, broccoli and sweet potato
    then put in steamer for 10 minutes.   If your shrimp or
    protein is frozen put it in with these items, otherwise
    wait until the last 3 minutes.
2. Prepare salad with lettuce, sliced radishes, radicchio
    and put in bowl
3. Prepare sauce with oils, nuts and nut butter, ginger,
    salt, coconut Aminos and apple cider vinegar (Note:
    coconut oil must be heated lightly to turn into liquid)
4. Spread steamed veggies on salad, then top with
    protein, then with avocado.
5. Top off all ingredients with sauce.

Chipotle Power Bowl

Ingredients for 1 Serving

Category 1) Raw Veggies

1. *Romaine Lettuce (or other lettuce) - handful*
2. *Sauerkraut - 1 tablespoon*
3. *Avocado - 1/2*
4. *Basil - 1/4 cup fresh (or 1 teaspoon dry)*
5. *1/2 lime*
6. *Sea Salt - a couple pinches or 1/2 teaspoon*
7. *Optional - Lemon Cilantro Dressing (or lemon, olive oil) 1 tablespoon*

Category 1) Steamed Veggies

1. *Cauliflower - 1/2 cup*
2. *Broccoli - 1/2 cup*

Category 2) Coconut Cream or Oil (optional: olive oil) 1-2 tablespoons

Category 3) Chipotle Lime Mayo (or other)

Category 5) Protein - Goat Cheese (or Chicken, Fish, Beef or Vegan Hemp Tofu) 2-3 oz.

Preparation

1. Chop and dice cauliflower and broccoli then put in steamer for 10 minutes.

2. Prepare salad with lettuce, basil, avocado
    and sauerkraut and put in bowl (add optional
    dressing)
3. Warm up coconut oil (Note: if you are cooking fish,
    chicken or beef sauté protein lightly over stove with
    coconut oil)
4. After 10 minutes, spread steamed veggies on salad,
    then top with protein, then with avocado.
5. Top off all ingredients with warm coconut oil, lime,
    chipotle mayo and salt.

Indian Soft Tacos

Ingredients for 1 Serving

Category 1) Raw Veggies

1. ***Butterleaf Lettuce (or other lettuce) - handful***
2. ***Raw sauerkraut - 1 large tablespoon***

Category 1) Steamed Veggies

1. ***Carrots - 1 small to medium sized***
2. ***Curry spice - 1 tablespoon***

Category 2) Walnut Oil (Coconut or Olive) - 1-2 tablespoons

Category 3) Nuts Almond Flour Tortilla (or Cassava, Coconut) - 1 tortilla

Category 4) Starch - Purple Yam (or sweet potato) - 1/4 cup chopped

Category 5) Protein - Organic Chicken (or Fish, Shrimp, Beef or Vegan Hemp Tofu) 2-3 oz.

Preparation

1. Chop and dice cauliflower, carrots and yams then put in steamer for 10 minutes.
2. Prepare salad with lettuce, sliced radishes, sauerkraut, 1/4 avocado, lemon and oil

3. Prepare protein with spice and oil and either steam or lightly sauté for 3-4 minutes
4. Heat up grain free tortilla for 1-2 minutes
5. Spread steamed veggies on tortilla with protein and spices and oil, spread left over onto salad
6. Top off taco with salt and lemon or lime

Mexican Taco Plate

Ingredients for 1 Serving

Category 1) Raw Veggies

1. ***Butterleaf Lettuce (or other lettuce) - handful***
2. ***Jicama - 1/3 cup***
3. ***Avocado - 1/2***
4. ***Lemon or Lime - 1/2***
5. ***Mexican Spice - 1 tablespoon***

Category 1) Steamed

1. ***Cauliflower Rice - 1/3 cup***
2. ***Swiss Chard - 1/2 cup***

Category 2) Olive Oil - 1-2 tablespoons

Category 3) Optional - Pecans or Pine Nuts - 1 handful

Category 4) Grain Free Tortillas - 2 shells

Category 5) Organic Grass Fed Cheese (or Beef, Chicken, Fish or Vegan Hemp Tofu) 2-3 oz.

Preparation

1. Chop salad and jicama and add to plate
2. Put avocado in separate bowl and use fork to mush into pulp
3. Add seasoning, olive oil, lemon or lime, and nuts to avocado to create guacamole
4. Optionally heat up taco shells for extra crispy texture

5. Add steamed veggies and optional protein to guacamole, stir and fill tacos
6. Add lettuce and jicama and grub down

Italian Sourdough Pizza Plate

Ingredients for 1 Serving

Category 1) Raw Veggies

1. ***Butterleaf Lettuce (or other lettuce) - handful***
2. ***Carrot - 1 medium size***
3. ***Avocado - 1/2***
4. ***Lemon - 1/2***
5. ***Marinara Sauce (organic) - 3/4 cup***

Category 2) Olive Oil - 1-2 tablespoons

Category 3) (optional) Pine nuts - 1 handful

Category 4) Fermented Sourdough - 1 slice

Category 5) Organic Grass Fed Cheese (or Beef or Vegan Hemp Tofu) 2-3 oz.

Preparation

1. Chop carrots, salad and avocado and add to plate
2. Cut cheese
3. Lightly heat marinara sauce (option to add beef, chicken or hemp tofu) 2-3 minutes
4. Toast slice of sourdough bread
5. Add cheese to sourdough and pour sauce on top
6. Add lemon and olive oil on top of both.

Banana Strawberry Coconut Avocado Smoothie

Ingredients for 7 Servings

Category 1) Raw Veggies & Fruits

1. *Avocados - 3 small or 2 large*
2. *Lemon or Lime - 7 regular size*
3. *Frozen organic strawberries - 1 cup*
4. *Raw Honey - 1 tablespoon*
5. *Water - 1-2 cups*
6. *Optional Spirulina Powder - 2-3 tablespoons*

Category 2) Coconut Cream 1/2 cup, Coconut or MTC Oil 2-3 tablespoons

Category 2 Option) 3-5 tablespoons of Raw Butter or Ghee from pasteurized grass fed cows

Category 3) 1 cup walnuts, almonds or macadamia (or combination)

Category 4) Frozen Green Bananas - 3 small or 2 large

Category 5) 7 Raw eggs or 1 cup whey protein

Category 5 Vegan Option) add additional tablespoon of spirulina and additional half cup of nuts

Preparation

1. Cut lemons and squeeze into blender (without seeds)
2. Add all other ingredients and blend. For thinner smoothie add more water.

3. Pour into separate mason jars and top off with lemon or lime for preservation.
4. Put into refrigerator and eat within 10 days
5. For lemon squeezer or mason jars go to our resources page HERE

Super Green Chocolate Tahini Butter Smoothie

Ingredients for 7 Servings

Category 1) Raw Veggies & Fruits

1. *Avocados - 3 small or 2 large*
2. *Lemon or Lime - 7 regular size*
3. *Raw Honey - 1 tablespoon*
4. *Water - 1-2 cups*
5. *Spirulina Powder - 2-3 tablespoons*
6. *Chocolate - 1 Bar (70% cacao or more)*

Category 2) 5-7 Tablespoons of Raw Grass Fed Butter or Ghee and/or 3-4 tablespoons Coconut or MTC Oil

Category 3) 1 cup walnuts, almonds or macadamia

Category 4) Frozen Green Bananas - 3 small or 2 large

Category 5) Raw eggs - 7 (option for vegan or whey protein - 1 cup)

Preparation

1. Cut lemons and squeeze into blender (without seeds)
2. Add all other ingredients and blend. For thinner smoothie add more water.
3. Pour into separate mason jars and top off with lemon for preservation.
4. Put into refrigerator and eat within 10 days
5. For lemon squeezer or mason jars go to our resources page HERE

Lemon Banana Ginger Turmeric Supersonic Smoothie

Ingredients for 7 Servings

Category 1) Raw Veggies & Fruits

1. *Avocados - 3 small or 2 large*
2. *Lemon or Lime - 7 regular size*
3. *Optional Raw Ginger and Turmeric - 1/3 cup of each*
4. *Raw Honey - 1 tablespoon*
5. *Water - 1-2 cups*
6. *Optional Spirulina Powder - 2-3 tablespoons*

Category 2) Coconut or MTC Oil 3-4 tablespoons

Category 2 Option) 5-7 tablespoons of Raw Butter or Ghee from pasteurized grass fed cows

Category 3) 1 cup walnuts, almonds or macadamia

Category 4) Frozen Green Bananas - 3 small or 2 large

Category 5) 7 Raw eggs or 1 cup whey protein

Category 5 Vegan Option) add additional tablespoon of spirulina and additional half cup of nuts

Preparation

1. Cut lemons and squeeze into blender (without seeds)
2. Add all other ingredients and blend. For thinner smoothie add more water.
3. Pour into separate mason jars and top off with lemon for preservation.
4. Put into refrigerator and eat within 10 days
5. For lemon squeezer or mason jars go to our resources page HERE

For more info or one-on-one coaching visit us here:
www.ChadScottCoaching.com

References

[1] https://www.ncbi.nlm.nih.gov/books/NBK279540/
[2] https://www.sciencedaily.com/releases/2019/07/190702112834.htm
[3] https://www.ncbi.nlm.nih.gov/pmc/articles/PMC2999748/
[4] https://www.webmd.com/heartburn-gerd/news/20170105/heartburn-drugs-may-raise-risk-of-stomach-infections-study#1
[5] https://www.ncbi.nlm.nih.gov/pmc/articles/PMC4656952/
[6] https://www.ncbi.nlm.nih.gov/pmc/articles/PMC5478398/
[7] https://www.jscimedcentral.com/CaseReports/casereports-1-1006.php
[8] https://www.who.int/news-room/fact-sheets/detail/obesity-and-overweight
[9] https://www.wvdhhr.org/bph/oehp/obesity/mortality.htm
[10] https://www.ncbi.nlm.nih.gov/pmc/articles/PMC1790820/
[11] https://www.obesityaction.org/community/article-library/obesity-and-type-2-diabetes
[12] https://www.ncbi.nlm.nih.gov/pmc/articles/PMC3109209/
[13] https://www.ncbi.nlm.nih.gov/pmc/articles/PMC4116271/
[14] https://www.health.harvard.edu/blog/200000-heart-disease-stroke-deaths-a-year-are-preventable-201309046648
[15] https://www.heart.org/en/get-involved/advocate/federal-priorities/cdc-prevention-programs
[16] https://pubmed.ncbi.nlm.nih.gov/29160902/
[17] https://www.cdc.gov/mmwr/volumes/69/wr/mm6915e3.htm
[18] Lisa S. Blackwell Columbia University Kali H. Trzesniewski and Carol Sorich Dweck. Implicit theories of intelligence predict achievement across an adolescent transition: a longitudinal study and an intervention. *Child Dev.* 2007 Jan-Feb;78(1):246-63. Stanford University

[19] https://www.ncbi.nlm.nih.gov/pmc/articles/PMC3463487/

[20] https://www.sciencedirect.com/science/article/abs/pii/S0031938414005095

[21] https://www.ncbi.nlm.nih.gov/pmc/articles/PMC2515351/

[22] https://www.ewg.org/research/timeline-bpa-invention-phase-out

[23] https://www.healthline.com/nutrition/nonstick-cookware-safety#section3

[24] https://www.ncbi.nlm.nih.gov/pmc/articles/PMC5672138/

[25] https://www.ncbi.nlm.nih.gov/pubmed/3899519

[26] https://www.nongmoproject.org/gmo-facts/

[27] https://www.ncbi.nlm.nih.gov/pubmed/9322581

[28] https://www.ncbi.nlm.nih.gov/pubmed/11759276

[29] https://www.ncbi.nlm.nih.gov/pubmed/17492525

[30] U.S. Department of Health and Human Services, Public Health Service, National Toxicology Program. 2005. 11th Report on Carcinogens.

[31] Sinha R, Rothman N, Brown ED, Salmon CP, Knize MG, Swanson CA, Rossi SC, Mark SD, Levander OA, Felton JS. High concentrations of the carcinogen 2-amino-1-methyl-6-phenylimidazo- [4,5-b]pyridine (PhIP) occur in chicken but are dependent on the cooking method. Cancer Res. 1995 Oct 15;55(20):4516-9.

[32] https://www.ncbi.nlm.nih.gov/pmc/articles/PMC6139832/

[33] https://www.ncbi.nlm.nih.gov/pmc/articles/PMC6139832/

[34] https://care.diabetesjournals.org/content/33/11/2477

[35] https://www.ncbi.nlm.nih.gov/pubmed/27934644

[36] https://www.ncbi.nlm.nih.gov/books/NBK22545/

[37] http://www.sciencedirect.com/science/article/pii/S0924224498000284

[38] https://www.ncbi.nlm.nih.gov/pubmed/29955693

[39] https://www.ncbi.nlm.nih.gov/pubmed/29955693

[40] https://www.ncbi.nlm.nih.gov/pmc/articles/PMC3685880/

[41] https://www.ncbi.nlm.nih.gov/pubmed/20396424

[42] https://www.ncbi.nlm.nih.gov/pubmed/25471197

[43] https://www.ncbi.nlm.nih.gov/pubmed/17998023

[44] https://www.ncbi.nlm.nih.gov/pubmed/27527212

[45] https://www.ncbi.nlm.nih.gov/pubmed/10499460

[46] https://www.ncbi.nlm.nih.gov/pubmed/27802855

[47] https://www.ncbi.nlm.nih.gov/pubmed/10073894

[48] https://www.ncbi.nlm.nih.gov/pubmed/19049813

[49] https://www.ncbi.nlm.nih.gov/pmc/articles/PMC3280075/

[50] https://www.ncbi.nlm.nih.gov/pubmed/2801588

[51] https://www.ncbi.nlm.nih.gov/pubmed/3354496

[52] https://www.ncbi.nlm.nih.gov/pubmed/15826055

[53] https://www.ncbi.nlm.nih.gov/pmc/articles/PMC6356561/

[54] http://onlinelibrary.wiley.com/doi/10.1111/j.1745-4549.2006.00092.x/abstract

[55] http://www.sciencedirect.com/science/article/pii/030881469290311O

[56] https://www.ncbi.nlm.nih.gov/pubmed/19774556
[57] https://www.ncbi.nlm.nih.gov/pubmed/22938099

[58] https://www.ncbi.nlm.nih.gov/pubmed/11453753

[59] http://www.tandfonline.com/doi/abs/10.1080/09540100220137655

[60] http://onlinelibrary.wiley.com/doi/10.1111/j.1365-2621.1983.tb14938.x/abstract

[61] https://www.ncbi.nlm.nih.gov/pubmed/15302522

[62] https://www.ncbi.nlm.nih.gov/pubmed/7001881

[63] https://www.hsph.harvard.edu/nutritionsource/anti-nutrients/lectins/

[64] https://www.ncbi.nlm.nih.gov/pmc/articles/PMC3426293/

[65] https://www.ncbi.nlm.nih.gov/pmc/articles/PMC1727292/

[66] https://www.ncbi.nlm.nih.gov/pmc/articles/PMC3705319/

[67] https://www.amymyersmd.com/2017/06/the-problem-with-grains-and-legumes/

[68] https://www.eurekalert.org/pub_releases/2016-10/sh-nsl101016.php

[69] https://www.ncbi.nlm.nih.gov/pmc/articles/PMC3406229/

[70] https://www.cdc.gov/mmwr/volumes/69/wr/mm6915e3.htm

[71] https://www.ncbi.nlm.nih.gov/pubmed/14673607

[72] http://pubs.acs.org/doi/abs/10.1021/jf072304b?

[73] https://www.ncbi.nlm.nih.gov/pmc/articles/PMC99017/

[74] https://www.ncbi.nlm.nih.gov/pmc/articles/PMC3195546/

[75] https://www.ncbi.nlm.nih.gov/pubmed/18950181

[76] Biochem. J. (1996) 317, 1–11 (Printed in Great Britain) 1 REVIEW ARTICLE The denaturation and degradation of stable enzymes at high temperatures Roy M. DANIEL*, Mark DINES and Helen H. PETACH† Department of Biological Sciences, The University of Waikato, Hamilton, New Zealand

[77] https://www.frontiersin.org/articles/10.3389/fpsyg.2018.00487/full

[78] Nutr Cancer. 2009; 61(4): 437–446.doi: Well-done Meat Intake, Heterocyclic Amine Exposure, and Cancer Risk Wei Zheng, M.D., Ph.D. and Sang-Ah Lee, Ph.D.

[79] Dungal (JAMA 176:788-08, 1961), Lijinsky and Shubik 9Science 143, 53-65, 1964)

[80] Food Funct. 2015 May;6(5):1684-91. doi: 10.1039/c5fo00251f. Differences and similarities in hepatic lipogenesis, gluconeogenesis and oxidative imbalance in mice fed diets rich in fructose or sucrose. Schultz A1, Barbosa-da-Silva S, Aguila MB, Mandarim-de-Lacerda CA.

[81] https://www.ncbi.nlm.nih.gov/pmc/articles/PMC2676420/
[82] https://www.ncbi.nlm.nih.gov/pubmed/27194405/

[83] https://www.ncbi.nlm.nih.gov/pubmed/18703413

[84] https://www.ncbi.nlm.nih.gov/pubmed/21418711

[85] https://www.ncbi.nlm.nih.gov/pubmed/23280226

[86] https://www.ncbi.nlm.nih.gov/pubmed/17263857

[87] https://www.ncbi.nlm.nih.gov/pmc/articles/PMC5651828/

[88] https://www.sciencedaily.com/releases/2014/02/140212093300.htm

[89] https://www.ncbi.nlm.nih.gov/pmc/articles/PMC6316842/

[90] https://www.ncbi.nlm.nih.gov/pmc/articles/PMC4105387/

[91] https://www.ncbi.nlm.nih.gov/pubmed/12594192

[92] https://onlinelibrary.wiley.com/doi/abs/10.1002/ijc.2910480517

[93] https://royalsocietypublishing.org/doi/10.1098/rsif.2017.0585

[94] https://www.ncbi.nlm.nih.gov/pmc/articles/PMC3263899/

[95] https://www.ncbi.nlm.nih.gov/pmc/articles/PMC4215472/

[96] https://www.ncbi.nlm.nih.gov/pmc/articles/PMC3752890/

[97] https://www.ncbi.nlm.nih.gov/pmc/articles/PMC3033553/

[98] https://www.ncbi.nlm.nih.gov/pmc/articles/PMC3056495/

[99] https://articles.mercola.com/sites/articles/archive/2020/09/06/travis-christofferson-nutritional-ketosis.aspx?

[100] https://www.ncbi.nlm.nih.gov/pmc/articles/PMC5025969/

[101] https://www.ncbi.nlm.nih.gov/pubmed/6099562

[102] http://www.nap.edu/read/10490/chapter/8#275

[103] https://www.ncbi.nlm.nih.gov/pubmed/17684196

[104] https://www.ncbi.nlm.nih.gov/pubmed/21489321

[105] https://www.ncbi.nlm.nih.gov/pubmed/22804876

[106] https://www.ncbi.nlm.nih.gov/pubmed/6538617

[107] https://www.ncbi.nlm.nih.gov/pubmed/17228046

[108] J. J. Meidenbauer, P. Mukherjee, and T. N. Seyfried, "The Glucose Ketone Index Calculator: A Simple Tool to Monitor Therapeutic Efficacy for Metabolic Management of Brain Cancer," Nutrition & Metabolism, vol. 12 (2015):12. DOI:10.1186/s12986-015-0009-2. Mercola, Joseph. Fat for Fuel (p. 304). Hay House. Kindle Edition.

[109] https://jamanetwork.com/journals/jama/fullarticle/2676543?alert=article

[110] https://www.health.harvard.edu/heart-health/are-eggs-risky-for-heart-health

[111] de Souza RJ , Mente A , Maroleanu A , et al. Intake of saturated and trans unsaturated fatty acids and risk of all cause mortality, cardiovascular disease, and type 2 diabetes:

systematic review and meta-analysis of observational
studies. BMJ 2015;351:h3978.doi:10.1136/bmj.h3978

[112]

http://www.ncbi.nlm.nih.gov/pubmed/20071648?itool=EntrezSystem2.PEntrez.Pubmed.Pub
med_ResultsPanel.Pubmed_RVDocSum&ordinalpos=2 Am J Clin Nutr.

[112] https://www.ncbi.nlm.nih.gov/pmc/articles/PMC5908176/

[113]

http://www.ncbi.nlm.nih.gov/pubmed?term=%22Archives+of+internal+medicine%22%5BJo
ur%5D+AND+1371%5Bpage%5D+AND+1992%5Bpdat%5D&cmd=detailssearch

[113] https://www.ncbi.nlm.nih.gov/pmc/articles/PMC5908176/

[114] https://www.ncbi.nlm.nih.gov/pmc/articles/PMC2755181/

[115] https://www.ncbi.nlm.nih.gov/pmc/articles/PMC5908176/

[116] https://www.ncbi.nlm.nih.gov/pmc/articles/PMC4299224/

[117] https://www.ncbi.nlm.nih.gov/pmc/articles/PMC4299224/

[118] https://www.ncbi.nlm.nih.gov/pmc/articles/PMC4433613/

[119] https://www.betterhealth.vic.gov.au/health/healthyliving/fats-and-oils

[120] https://www.ncbi.nlm.nih.gov/pmc/articles/PMC6140086/#__sec2title

[121] https://www.ncbi.nlm.nih.gov/pmc/articles/PMC3335257/

[122] https://www.ncbi.nlm.nih.gov/pubmed/12442909

[123] https://www.ncbi.nlm.nih.gov/pmc/articles/PMC3253931/

[124] https://www.sciencedaily.com/releases/2019/12/191211171335.htm

[125] http://www.cell.com/cell/fulltext/S0092-8674(16)30972-2

[126] https://www.ncbi.nlm.nih.gov/pubmed/17445348

[127] https://www.ncbi.nlm.nih.gov/pubmed/26151029/

[128] https://www.ncbi.nlm.nih.gov/pubmed/9772143

[129] Morton RW, Murphy KT, McKellar SR, Schoenfield BJ, Henselmans M, Helms E,
Aragon AA, Devries MC, Banfield L, Krieger JW, Phillips SM. A systematic review, meta-
analysis and meta-regression of the effect of protein supplementation on resistance
training-induced gains in muscle mass and strength in healthy adults. *Br J Sports
Med.* 2018 Mar;52(6):376-84.

[130] Thomas DT, Erdman KA, Burke LM. Position of the Academy of Nutrition and Dietetics,
Dietitians of Canada, and the American College of Sports Medicine: Nutrition and athletic
performance. *J Acad Nutr Diet.* 2016 Mar;116(3):501-28.

[131] Berryman CE, Lieberman HR, Fulgoni VL, Pasiakos SM. Protein intake trends and conformity with the Dietary Reference Intakes in the United States: Analysis of the National Health and Nutrition Examination Survey, 2001–2014. *Am J Clin Nutr.* 2018 Aug;108(2):405-13.

[132] https://www.ncbi.nlm.nih.gov/pmc/articles/PMC3197704/

[133] Dietary Reference Intakes for energy, carbohydrate, fiber, fat, fatty acids, cholesterol, protein, and amino acids. Washington, D.C.: National Academy Press; 2005.

[134] https://www.sciencedaily.com/releases/2017/09/170914084035.htm

[135] https://www.ncbi.nlm.nih.gov/pmc/articles/PMC1480571/

[136] M. I. Frisard et al., "Effect of 6-Month Calorie Restriction on Biomarkers of Longevity, Metabolic Adaptation, and Oxidative Stress in Overweight Individuals: A Randomized Controlled Trial," http://jamanetwork.com/journals/jama/fullarticle/1108368. Mercola, Joseph. Fat for Fuel (p. 306). Hay House. Kindle Edition.

[137] M. E. Levine et al., "Low Protein Intake Is Associated with a Major Reduction in IGF-1, Cancer, and Overall Mortality in the 65 and Younger but Not Older Population," Cell Metabolism, 19, no. 3 (2014): 407–17, DOI: 10.1016/j .cmet.2014.02.006.

[138] https://www.frontiersin.org/articles/10.3389/fendo.2019.00142/full

[139] Janeiro MH, Ramírez MJ, Milagro FI, Martínez JA, Solas M. Implication of trimethylamine N-oxide (TMAO) in disease: Potential biomarker or new therapeutic target. *Nutrients.* 2018 Oct;10(10):1398.

[140] Li Z, Wong A, Henning SM, Zhang Y, Jones A, Zerlin A, Thames G, Bowerman S, Tseng CH, Heber D. Hass avocado modulates postprandial vascular reactivity and postprandial inflammatory responses to a hamburger meal in healthy volunteers. *Food Funct.* 2013 Feb;4(3):384-91.

[141] Rizzo NS, Jaceldo-Siegl K, Sabate J, Fraser GE. Nutrient profiles of vegetarian and nonvegetarian dietary patterns. *J Acad Nutr Diet.* 2013 Dec;113(12):1610-9.

[142] National Research Council (US) Subcommittee on the Tenth Edition of the Recommended Dietary Allowances. Washington (DC): National Academies Press (US); 1989.

[143] Young VR, Pellett PL. Plant proteins in relation to human protein and amino acid nutrition. *Am J Clin Nutr.* 1994 May;59(5 Suppl):1203S-12S.

[144] McDougall J. Plant foods have a complete amino acid composition. *Circulation.* 2002 Jun;105(25):e197.

[145] http://nutritiondata.self.com/facts/vegetables-and-vegetable-products/2765/2

[146] https://www.ncbi.nlm.nih.gov/pmc/articles/PMC2730948/

[147] Reidy PT, Rasmussen BB. Role of ingested amino acids and protein in the promotion of resistance exercise–induced muscle protein anabolism. *J Nutr.* 2016 Feb;146(2):155-83.

[148] https://academic.oup.com/biomedgerontology/advance-article/doi/10.1093/gerona/gly201/5106141

[149] https://www.eatright.org/fitness/sports-and-performance/fueling-your-workout/protein-and-the-athlete

[150] http://pubs.rsc.org/en/content/articlehtml/2016/fo/c5fo01530h

[151] https://www.ncbi.nlm.nih.gov/pmc/articles/PMC3572016/

[152] https://jasn.asnjournals.org/content/28/1/304.abstract

[153] https://www.cdc.gov/nchs/data/factsheets/factsheet_nhanes.htm

[154] https://www.niddk.nih.gov/health-information/digestive-diseases/digestive-system-how-it-works

[155] https://www.aan.com/PressRoom/home/PressRelease/1023

[156] https://www.ncbi.nlm.nih.gov/pmc/articles/PMC5952217/

[157] https://www.ncbi.nlm.nih.gov/pmc/articles/PMC2127586/

[158] https://www.ncbi.nlm.nih.gov/pubmed/17929537

[159] https://www.ncbi.nlm.nih.gov/pubmed/17306982

[160] https://www.ncbi.nlm.nih.gov/pubmed/10398297

[161] https://www.ncbi.nlm.nih.gov/pubmed/23244540

[162] https://www.ncbi.nlm.nih.gov/pmc/articles/PMC5394735/

[163] https://www.ncbi.nlm.nih.gov/pmc/articles/PMC5783752/

[164] https://www.ncbi.nlm.nih.gov/pubmed/25201001

[165] https://www.ncbi.nlm.nih.gov/pubmed/18224538

[166] https://www.ncbi.nlm.nih.gov/pubmed/25201001

[167] https://en.wikipedia.org/wiki/Diminishing_returns

[168] https://www.nature.com/articles/s41467-019-13540-4

[169] https://www.ncbi.nlm.nih.gov/pmc/articles/PMC4388596/

[170] https://www.ncbi.nlm.nih.gov/pmc/articles/PMC3106288/

[171] https://www.tandfonline.com/doi/abs/10.4161/auto.6.6.12376

[172] https://academic.oup.com/jcem/article-abstract/74/4/757/3004645?redirectedFrom=fulltext

[173] https://www.ncbi.nlm.nih.gov/pmc/articles/PMC3463459/
[174] https://onlinelibrary.wiley.com/doi/abs/10.1002/ejsp.674

[175] https://academic.oup.com/ajcn/article-abstract/26/11/1180/4732762

[176] https://newsroom.heart.org/news/gobbling-your-food-may-harm-your-waistline-and-heart

[177] https://www.ncbi.nlm.nih.gov/pubmed/21802566

[178] https://www.health.harvard.edu/newsletter_article/stress-and-the-sensitive-gut

[179] https://www.niddk.nih.gov/health-information/digestive-diseases/acid-reflux-ger-gerd-adults/symptoms-causes

[180] https://www.sciencedaily.com/releases/2012/01/120118111740.htm

[181] https://onlinelibrary.wiley.com/doi/full/10.1002/oby.20460

[182] https://www.tandfonline.com/doi/abs/10.3109/07853899009148930

[183] Kris-Etherton P, Taylor DS, Yu-Poth S, et al. Polyunsaturated fatty acids in the food chain in the United States. Am J Clin Nutr. 2000;71(1):179S-188S. doi:10.1093/ajcn/71.1.179S.

[184] Swanson D, Block R, Mousa SA. Omega-3 fatty acids EPA and DHA: health benefits throughout life. Adv Nutr. 2012;3(1):1-7. doi:10.3945/an.111.000893; Nkondjock A, Ghadirian P. Intake of specific carotenoids and essential fatty acids and breast cancer risk in Montreal, Canada. Am J Clin Nutr. 2004;79(5):857-864. doi:10.1093/ajcn/79.5.857.

[185] Parker G, Gibson NA, Brotchie H, Heruc G, Rees A-M, Hadzi-Pavlovic D. Omega-3 Fatty Acids and Mood Disorders. Am J Psychiatry. 2006;163(6):969-978. doi:10.1176/ajp.2006.163.6.969; Logan AC. Omega-3 fatty acids and major depression: a primer for the mental health professional. Lipids Health Dis. 2004;3:25. doi:10.1186/1476-511X-3-25; Kiecolt-Glaser JK, Belury MA, Andridge R, Malarkey WB, Glaser R. Omega-3 supplementation lowers inflammation and anxiety in medical students: a randomized controlled trial. Brain Behav Immun. 2011;25(8):1725-1734. doi:10.1016/j.bbi.2011.07.229.

[186] Kalmijn S, van Boxtel MPJ, Ocké M, Verschuren WMM, Kromhout D, Launer LJ. Dietary intake of fatty acids and fish in relation to cognitive performance at middle age. Neurology. 2004;62(2):275-280.

[187] Goldberg RJ, Katz J. A meta-analysis of the analgesic effects of omega-3 polyunsaturated fatty acid supplementation for inflammatory joint pain. Pain. 2007;129(1):210-223. doi:10.1016/j.pain.2007.01.020.

[188] Couet C, Delarue J, Ritz P, Antoine JM, Lamisse F. Effect of dietary fish oil on body fat mass and basal fat oxidation in healthy adults. Int J Obes Relat Metab Disord. 1997;21(8):637-643.

[189] Buckley JD, Howe PRC. Anti-obesity effects of long-chain omega-3 polyunsaturated fatty acids. Obes Rev. 2009;10(6):648-659. doi:10.1111/j.1467-789X.2009.00584.x.

[190] Smith GI, Atherton P, Reeds DN, et al. Omega-3 polyunsaturated fatty acids augment the muscle protein anabolic response to hyperinsulinaemia–hyperaminoacidaemia in healthy young and middle-aged men and women. Clin Sci. 2011;121(6):267-278. doi:10.1042/CS20100597.

[191] https://corpus.ulaval.ca/jspui/bitstream/20.500.11794/15362/1/effect_of_lactobacillus_rhamnosus_cgmcc13724_supplementation_on_weight_loss_and_maintenance_in_obese_men_and_women.pdf

[192] http://saveoursoils.com/userfiles/downloads/1351255687-Changes%20in%20USDA%20food%20composition%20data%20for%2043%20garden%20crops,%201950-1999.pdf

[193] Holick MF. Vitamin D is essential to the modern indoor lifestyle. Science News Website. https://www.sciencenews.org/article/vitamin-d-essential-modern-indoor-lifestyle. October 8, 2010. Accessed August 26, 2018; Holick MF. Vitamin D: evolutionary, physiological and health perspectives. Curr Drug Targets. 2011;12(1):4-18. 50. Wacker M, Holick MF. Vitamin D - effects on skeletal and extraskeletal health and the need for supplementation. Nutrients. 2013;5(1):111-148. doi:10.3390/nu5010111. 51. Dawson-Hughes B, Mithal A, Bonjour J-P, et al. IOF position statement: vitamin D recommendations for older adults. Osteoporos Int. 2010;21(7):1151-1154. doi:10.1007/

[194] Dawson-Hughes B, Mithal A, Bonjour J-P, et al. IOF position statement: vitamin D recommendations for older adults. Osteoporos Int. 2010;21(7):1151-1154. doi:10.1007/s00198-010-1285-3; Wang TJ, Pencina MJ, Booth SL, et al. Vitamin D Deficiency and Risk of Cardiovascular Disease. Circulation. 2008;117(4):503-511. doi:10.1161/CIRCULATIONAHA.107.706127; Pilz S, Dobnig H, Fischer JE, et al. Low Vitamin D Levels Predict Stroke in Patients Referred to Coronary Angiography. Stroke. 2008;39(9):2611-2613. doi:10.1161/STROKEAHA.107.513655; Giovannucci E. Epidemiological Evidence for Vitamin D and Colorectal Cancer. J Bone Miner Res. 2007;22(S2):V81-V85. doi:10.1359/jbmr.07s206; Hyppönen E, Läärä E, Reunanen A, Järvelin M-R, Virtanen SM. Intake of vitamin D and risk of type 1 diabetes: a birth-cohort study. Lancet. 2001;358(9292):1500-1503. doi:10.1016/S0140-6736(01)06580-1; Munger KL, Levin LI, Hollis BW, Howard NS, Ascherio A. Serum 25-Hydroxyvitamin D Levels and Risk of Multiple Sclerosis. JAMA. 2006;296(23):2832. doi:10.1001/jama.296.23.2832; Nnoaham KE, Clarke A. Low serum vitamin D levels and tuberculosis: a systematic review and meta-analysis. Int J Epidemiol. 2008;37(1):113-119. doi:10.1093/ije/dym247; Cannell JJ, Vieth R, Umhau JC, et al. Epidemic influenza and vitamin D. Epidemiol Infect. 2006;134(06):1129. doi:10.1017/S0950268806007175.

[195] Holick MF. Vitamin D: importance in the prevention of cancers, type 1 diabetes, heart disease, and osteoporosis. Am J Clin Nutr. 2004;79(3):362-371. doi:10.1093/ajcn/79.3.362.

[196] Norman, A. W. (2008). From vitamin D to hormone D: fundamentals of the vitamin D endocrine system essential for good health. The American Journal of Clinical Nutrition, 88(2), 491S-499S.

[197] Tomlinson, P. B., Joseph, C., & Angioi, M. (2015). Effects of vitamin D supplementation on upper and lower body muscle strength levels in healthy individuals. A systematic review with meta-analysis. Journal of Science and Medicine in Sport, 18(5), 575-580.

[198] https://www.ncbi.nlm.nih.gov/pubmed/18419308

[199] https://www.ncbi.nlm.nih.gov/pubmed/18337721/

[200] http://www.jneurosci.org/content/20/9/3139.short

[201] https://www.ncbi.nlm.nih.gov/pmc/articles/PMC4487780/

[202] https://www.sciencedirect.com/science/article/pii/S0092867407009737

[203] https://science.sciencemag.org/content/350/6265/1208.full

[204] https://www.sciencedirect.com/science/article/pii/S0092867408008799

[205] https://www.ncbi.nlm.nih.gov/pubmed/21937766

[206] https://science.sciencemag.org/content/342/6158/1243417

[207] https://www.sciencedirect.com/science/article/pii/B9780120354115500071

[208] https://www.sciencedirect.com/science/article/abs/pii/S0306452206016617

[209] https://iubmb.onlinelibrary.wiley.com/doi/abs/10.1080/152165401753311780

[210] https://link.springer.com/article/10.1007/s11010-010-0391-z

[211] https://www.sciencedirect.com/science/article/pii/S0092867407009737

[212] https://journals.plos.org/plosone/article?id=10.1371/journal.pone.0042357

[213] https://www.sciencedirect.com/science/article/pii/S0924857920300984#bib0069

[214] https://www.ncbi.nlm.nih.gov/pmc/articles/PMC4915787/

[215] https://www.sciencedaily.com/releases/2001/10/011011065609.htm

[216] https://www.sciencedirect.com/science/article/abs/pii/S1756464619300313?via%3Dihub

[217] https://www.medicalnewstoday.com/articles/323288

[218] https://www.ncbi.nlm.nih.gov/pmc/articles/PMC353050/

[219] https://journals.plos.org/plospathogens/article?id=10.1371/journal.ppat.1001176

[220] https://www.ncbi.nlm.nih.gov/pubmed/19260845

[221] https://www.ncbi.nlm.nih.gov/pubmed/18784609

[222] https://www.ncbi.nlm.nih.gov/pubmed/12472620

[223] https://www.ncbi.nlm.nih.gov/pubmed/19781622

[224] https://www.ncbi.nlm.nih.gov/pubmed/18801111

[225] https://www.ncbi.nlm.nih.gov/pubmed/20691074

[226] Groeneveld GJ, Beijer C, Veldink JH, Kalmijn S, Wokke JHJ, van den Berg LH. Few Adverse Effects of Long-Term Creatine Supplementation in a Placebo-Controlled Trial. Int J Sports Med. 2005;26(4):307-313. doi:10.1055/s-2004-817917.

[227] Branch JD. Effect of creatine supplementation on body composition and performance: a meta-analysis. Int J Sport Nutr Exerc Metab. 2003;13(2):198-226.

[228] Volek JS, Ratamess NA, Rubin MR, et al. The effects of creatine supplementation on muscular performance and body composition responses to short-term resistance training overreaching. Eur J Appl Physiol. 2004;91(5-6):628-637. doi:10.1007/s00421-003-1031-z.

[229] Eckerson JM, Stout JR, Moore GA, et al. Effect of Creatine Phosphate Supplementation on Anaerobic Working Capacity and Body Weight After Two and Six Days of Loading in Men and Women. J Strength Cond Res. 2005;19(4):756. doi:10.1519/R-16924.1.

[230] Bassit RA, Pinheiro CH da J, Vitzel KF, Sproesser AJ, Silveira LR, Curi R. Effect of short-term creatine supplementation on markers of skeletal muscle damage after strenuous contractile.

[231] Darrabie MD, Arciniegas AJL, Mishra R, Bowles DE, Jacobs DO, Santacruz L. AMPK and substrate availability regulate creatine transport in cultured cardiomyocytes. Am J Physiol Metab. 2011;300(5):E870-E876. doi:10.1152/ajpendo.00554.2010; Guzun R, Timohhina N, Tepp K, et al. Systems bioenergetics of creatine kinase networks: physiological roles of creatine and phosphocreatine in regulation of cardiac cell function. Amino Acids. 2011;40(5):1333-1348. doi:10.1007/s00726-011-0854-x.

[232] Parise G, Mihic S, MacLennan D, Yarasheski KE, Tarnopolsky MA. Effects of acute creatine monohydrate supplementation on leucine kinetics and mixed-muscle protein synthesis. J Appl Physiol. 2001;91(3):1041-1047. doi:10.1152/jappl.2001.91.3.1041; Safdar A, Yardley NJ, Snow R, Melov S, Tarnopolsky MA. Global and targeted gene expression and protein content in skeletal muscle of young men following short-term creatine monohydrate supplementation. Physiol Genomics. 2008;32(2):219-228. doi:10.1152/physiolgenomics.00157.2007. Matthews, Michael. Bigger Leaner Stronger: The Simple Science of Building the Ultimate Male Body (Muscle for Life Book 1) (p. 484). Oculus Publishers. Kindle Edition.

[233] Perez-Guisado J, Jakeman PM. Citrulline Malate Enhances Athletic Anaerobic Performance and Relieves Muscle Soreness. J Strength Cond Res. 2010;24(5);1215:1222. Doi:10:1519/JSC.0b0l3e3181cb28el).
[234] Bescos R Surenda A. Tur JA, Pons A. The Effect of Nitric-Oxide-Related Supplements on Human Performance. Sport Med. 2012:42(2):99-117. Doi:10.2165/11596860-00000000-00000; Orozco-Gutiérrez JJ, Castillo-Martinez L. Orea-Tejeda A, et al. Effect of L-arginine or L-citrulline oral supplementation on blood pressure and right ventricular functions in heart failure patients with preserved erection fraction. Cardiol J. 2010;17(6):612-618; Cormio L, De Siati M, Lorusso F, et al. Oral L-Citrulline Supplementation Improved Erection Hardness in Men With Mild Erectile Dysfunction. Urology. 20111;77(1):119-112. Doi:10.1016fj. urology.2010.08.028.
[235] https://www.ncbi.nlm.nih.gov/pmc/articles/PMC4989512/
[236] https://www.ncbi.nlm.nih.gov/pmc/articles/PMC2905334/

[237] https://www.afcpe.org/news-and-publications/the-standard/2018-3/the-power-of-accountability/